Neuroradiology - Images vs Symptoms

Martina Špero • Hrvoje Vavro

Neuroradiology - Images vs Symptoms

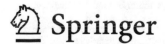 Springer

Martina Špero
Diagnostic and Interventional Radiology
Clinical Hospital Dubrava
Zagreb
Croatia

Hrvoje Vavro
Diagnostic and Interventional Radiology
Clinical Hospital Dubrava
Zagreb
Croatia

ISBN 978-3-030-69215-5   ISBN 978-3-030-69213-1   (eBook)
https://doi.org/10.1007/978-3-030-69213-1

This Springer imprint is published by the registered company Springer Nature Switzerland AG
The registered company address is: Gewerbestrasse 11, 6330 Cham, Switzerland

Acknowledgements

After our first book, *Neuroradiology: Expect the Unexpected*, has proved to be a success, we decided we have more to say. Therefore, here we are again, speaking out about rare neuroradiological pathologies and problems we faced while trying to report them accurately.

The concept of this book, titled *Neuroradiology: Images vs Symptoms*, is a little bit different compared to the first one. The content is divided into three sections according to the leading symptoms our patients presented with in hospital emergency units or as outpatients. Our intention was to emphasize two facts. First, rare and serious conditions could be hidden behind common (mis)leading neurological symptoms. Second, it is important to collaborate with clinician colleagues because neuroradiologist needs complete and accurate patient information to make a proper diagnosis or a differential diagnosis which could direct further diagnostic processing in the right direction.

Cases we have prepared this time are rare and peculiar cases, or usual cases with a twist from our everyday practice. Those cases proved to be a surprise for us in a way, although we are both neuroradiologist with almost two decades of experience. This book was created during a challenging times marked by pandemic of the new virus and severe earthquake that struck Zagreb, the capital of Croatia, and the city where we live and work. Such difficult times and situations affect each of us and change us in different ways. Despite the difficult times, we hope that once again, we have together managed to create a book you will enjoy reading. We also hope this book will be helpful to our readers in solving future cases.

We would like to thank Antonella Cerri from Springer Italy who supported our wish to contribute again with this book and wrote about neuroradiology, the part of radiology in which we really enjoy.

We wish to thank Boris Brkljačić, professor of radiology and the chairman of our department, who always supported our work.

Special thanks to all our colleagues from Croatia and abroad for being our friends and teachers and for supporting us and our work over many years.

We are immensely grateful to the closest members of our families, to our closest friends and colleagues, who always stood by us, helping us and supporting us in our private and professional lives. We are also grateful to those closest to us who showed understanding and gave us time and space to create this publication despite all the other private and business obligations.

Zagreb, Croatia   Martina Špero
                                                                         Hrvoje Vavro

Contents

Abbreviations

β-HCG	β-chorionic gonadotropin
Ab	Antibody
ADAMTS13	ADAM Metallopeptidase with Thrombospondin Type 1 Motif 13
ADC	Apparent diffusion coefficient
AFP	α-fetoprotein
AIDS	Acquired immunodeficiency syndrome
AILE	Autoimmune limbic encephalitis
AML	Acute myeloid leukemia
AN	Anorexia nervosa
CAPNON	Calcifying pseudoneoplasm of the neuraxis
CAR	Chimeric antigen receptor
CASPR2	Contactin-associated protein-2
CBM	Converted bone marrow
CBV	Cerebral blood volume
CISS	Constructive interference in steady-state
CJD	Creutzfeldt–Jakob disease
CLL	Chronic lymphocytic leukaemia
CM	Cavernous malformation
CNS	Central nervous system
CSF	Cerebrospinal fluid
CT	Computed tomography
CTA	Computed tomography angiography
DNA	Deoxyribonucleic acid
DSA	Digital subtraction angiography
DVA	Developmental venous abnormality
DWI	Diffusion weighted imaging
EHD	Emergency hospital department
EMG	Electromyelography
ESM	Extradural spinal meningioma
FDG	Fluorodeoxyglucose
FLAIR	Fluid attenuation inversion recovery
FS	Fat suppressed
FSE	Fast spin echo
GCT	Germ cell tumor
GEOS	Genetics of early onset stroke
GTR	Gross total resection

HAART	Highly active antiretroviral therapy
HBV	Hepatitis B virus
HCV	Hepatitis C virus
HU	Hounsfield units
HUS	Haemolytic-uremic syndrome
ICH	Intracerebral haematoma
IDH	Isocitrate dehydrogenase
IVF	In vitro fertilization
IVM	Intraventricular meningioma
JCV	John Cunningham virus
LGI-1	Leucine-rich glioma inactivated 1
MAHA	Microangiopathic haemolytic anaemia
MBD	Mineral bone density
MRA	Magnetic resonance angiography
MRI	Magnetic resonance imaging
MRS	Magnetic resonance spectroscopy
MS	Myeloid sarcoma
MT	Mature teratoma
MVNT	Multinodular and vacuolating neuronal tumour
NAA	N-acetyl aspartate
NMDA	N-methyl-D-aspartate
PET	Positron emission tomography
PNS	Peripheral nervous system
rCBV	Relative cerebral blood volume
rtPA	Recombinant tissue plasminogen activator
SEAC	Spinal extradural arachnoid cyst
STIR	Short tau inversion recovery
SWI	Susceptibility weighted imaging
TIRM	Turbo inversion recovery magnitude
TMA	Thrombotic microangiopathy
TN	Trigeminal neuralgia
TPE	Therapeutic plasma exchange
TTP	Thrombotic thrombocytopenic purpura
VGCC	Voltage-gated calcium channel
VGKC	Voltage-gated potassium channel
VRT	Volume rendering technique
VWF	Von Willebrand factor
WHO	World Health Organization

Part I

Pain and Vertigo

Voltage-Gated Potassium Channel (VGKC)-Complex Antibody Limbic Encephalitis

In the second half of January 2019, a 46-year-old male patient was hospitalized due to electrolyte disorder: hypokalaemia (2.7 mmol/L; normal levels 3.9–5.1 mmol/L) and hyponatraemia (100 mmol/L; normal levels 137–146 mmol/L). The patient was former alcoholic and smoker and on antihypertensive therapy including diuretic (perindopril and indapamide). During the previous week the patient had flu-like symptoms, he was weak, febrile, coughing and vomiting and did not have appetite.

The night before hospitalization, the patient had headache and vertigo, was restless, confused and collapsed on one occasion. Therefore, he was brought to our hospital: on admission, head CT was reported normal (Fig. 1.1), the patient was afebrile, white blood cell count and C-reactive protein were slightly elevated, chest X-ray did not reveal lung infiltration.

The patient was hospitalised due to low potassium and sodium levels at first presumed to be a result of vomiting and diuretic therapy. Nasopharyngeal swab was positive for influenza virus A. Chest CT confirmed bilateral ground-glass opacities with small consolidations in peripheral parts of all lung lobes indicating pneumonia. He was treated with oseltamivir for flu and levofloxacin for pneumonia. Electrolyte disorder was treated with hypertonic saline at first, later on with fluid and electrolyte replacement. Applied therapy resulted in normal values of inflammatory parameters in 5 days and normal levels of sodium and potassium in 7 days.

While his overall condition was gradually getting better, our patient became disoriented, agitated and logorrheic with tremor and left hand dysmetria. Brain MRI was performed 4 days after the admission and was reported by general radiologist (Fig. 1.2). The second MRI was performed 19 days after the admission, at the beginning of February, and was reported by neuroradiologist (Fig. 1.3). Clinician referral for both brain MRI was central pontine myelinolysis.

Regarding clinician referral, pons was normal in size and signal intensities in all sequences on both MRI. In comparison to the first MRI, neuroradiologist considered that described changes already existed on the initial brain MRI (Fig. 1.2), but were less pronounced and not recognized by general radiologist.

While reporting the second MRI, due to clinical data on metabolic changes neuroradiologist has suspected possible extrapontine myelinolysis or limbic encephalitis.

Chest and abdominal CT were performed to exclude possible paraneoplastic syndrome, which did not reveal neoplastic process, and tumour markers were within the normal range. Thyroid hormones were within the normal range, but serum vitamin B_{12} level was low, indicating B_{12} hypovitaminosis. CSF analysis revealed increased

M. Špero, H. Vavro, *Neuroradiology - Images vs Symptoms*,
https://doi.org/10.1007/978-3-030-69213-1_1

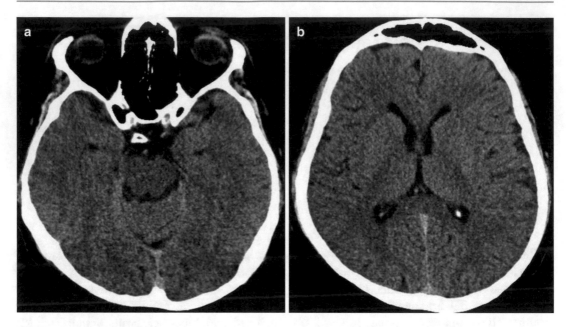

Fig. 1.1 Computed tomography of the brain, axial scans (**a**, **b**), performed on admission: reported normal

protein level 0.46 g/L (0.17–0.37 g/L) and lactate dehydrogenase level 34 U/L (<24 U/L).

Psychiatrists and neurologists were consulted, but their reports were inconclusive.

After the second MRI, one of the attending neurologists suspected possible autoimmune encephalitis could be the cause of the patient symptoms and MRI changes. Only anti-VGKC Ab in serum was elevated, 100 pmol/L (normal level <85 pmol/L), while serum NMDA-receptor Ab, LGI-1 Ab, CASPR2 Ab, anti-VGCC (PQ-type) Ab and anti-VGCC (N-type) Ab were negative. Serum Hu, Yo, Ri antibodies were negative as well. CSF anti-VGKC Ab was normal 13.4 pmol/L (<85 pmol/L), as well as CSF NMDA receptor, LGI-1, CASPR2 antibodies.

Psychiatric symptoms improved to benzodiazepine therapy, while neurological symptoms persisted.

In May 2019 anti-VGKC Ab level increased (150 pmol/L), LGI-1 and CASPR2 antibodies

were negative. Follow-up brain MRI revealed bilateral volume reduction of amygdala, hippocampus, putamen, nucleus caudatus and medial globus pallidus, T2WI and FLAIR signal intensities were still slightly increased, and linear cortical hyperintensity in dorsal part of right precentral gyrus was decreased in size and signal intensity (Fig. 1.4). SWI revealed hypointense putamen and globus pallidus on both sides, probably due to degenerative changes in the process of autoimmune encephalitis (Fig. 1.5).

After pulse corticosteroid therapy in May neurological symptoms persisted, but have improved for a short period of time after intravenous immunoglobulin therapy in July 2019. Rituximab therapy was initiated in July 2019 due to increased anti-VGKC AB level (360 pmol/L) without changes in neurological symptoms. After several monoclonal antibody treatment cycle, anti-VGKC AB levels were within the normal range or elevated up to 120 pmol/L, left hand dysmetria

Fig. 1.2 Brain MRI 4 days after the admission, axial T2WI (**a–c**) and FLAIR (**d–f**), reported by general radiologist who reported one small gliotic lesion in subcorti-

cal white matter in both frontal lobes, the rest was, according to attending radiologist, unremarkable

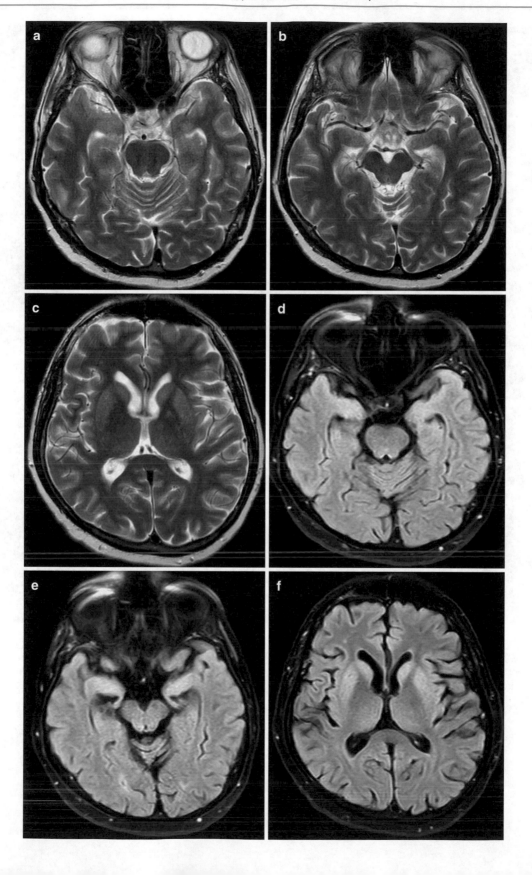

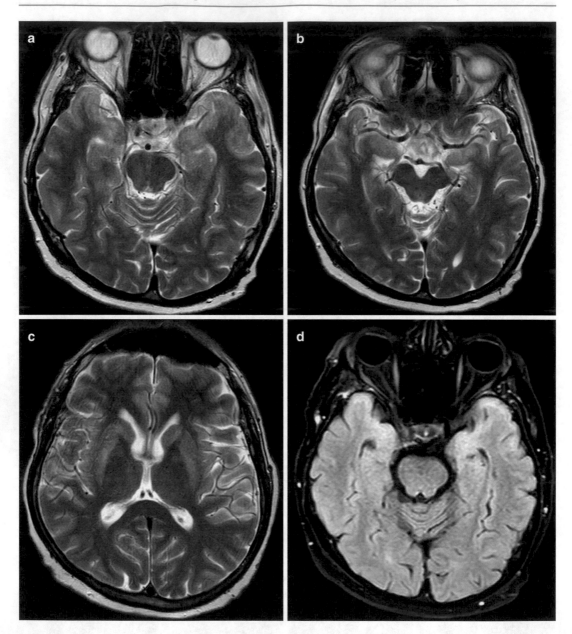

Fig. 1.3 Brain MRI 19 days after the admission, axial T2WI (**a–c**, **g**, **h**), FLAIR FS (**d–f**, **j**, **k**) DWI (**i**), ADC (**l**), reported by neuroradiologist. Bilateral T2WI and FLAIR FS hyperintensities of putamen, nucleus caudatus and medial part of globus pallidus, hyperintense were cortex of hippocampus and amygdala on both sides and dorsal part of right precentral gyrus. DWI and ADC did not reveal restricted diffusion, although basal ganglia seemed discreetly hyperintense on DWI. Involved structures were hypointense on T1WI, without contrast enhancement on post-contrast MRI, and did not increase in volume

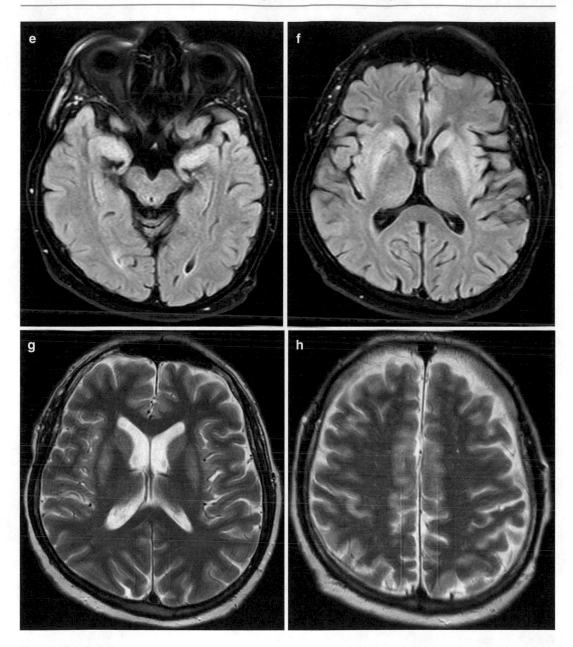

Fig. 1.3 (continued)

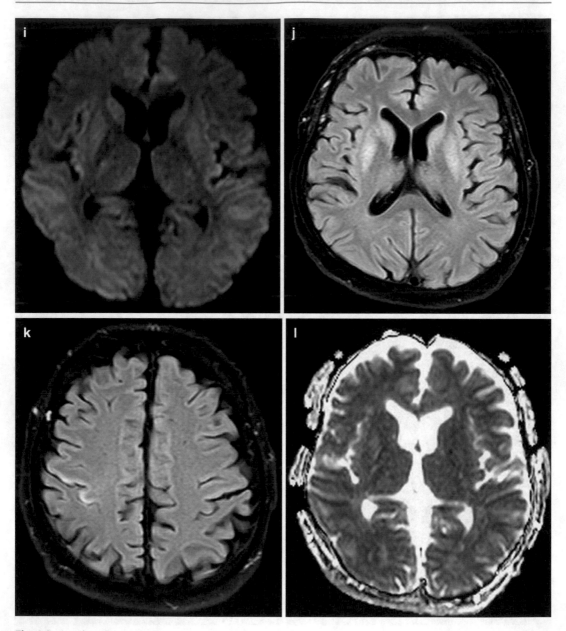

Fig. 1.3 (continued)

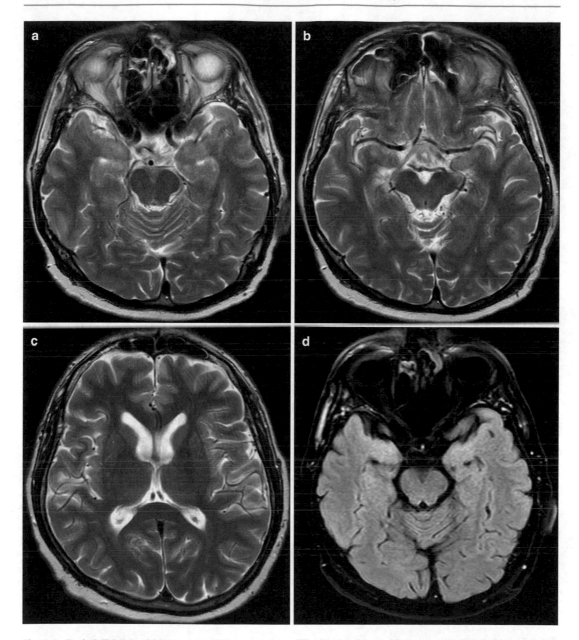

Fig. 1.4 Brain MRI (May 2019), axial T2WI (**a–c, g, h**), FLAIR FS (**d–f, j, k**) DWI (**i**), ADC (**l**) revealed bilateral amygdala, hippocampus, putamen, nucleus caudatus and medial globus pallidus volume reduction, T2WI and FLAIR signal intensities were still slightly increased, linear cortical hyperintensity in dorsal part of right precentral gyrus was decreasing in size and signal intensity

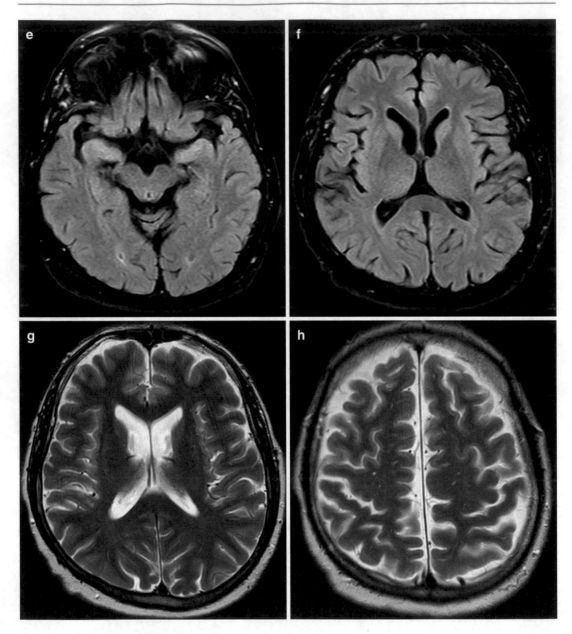

Fig. 1.4 (continued)

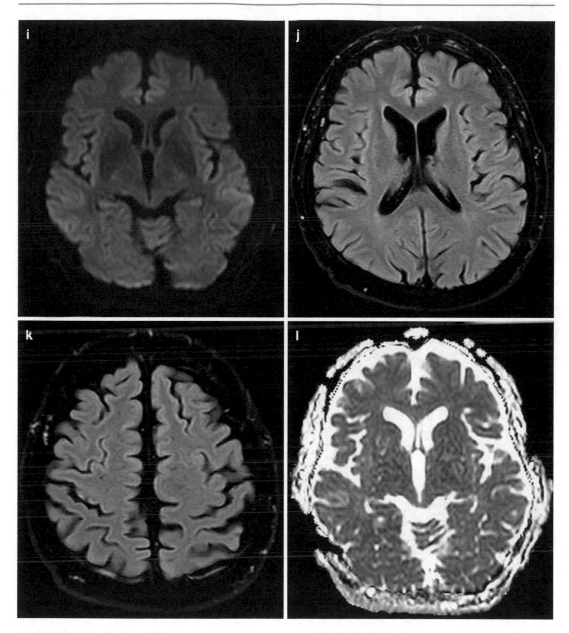

Fig. 1.4 (continued)

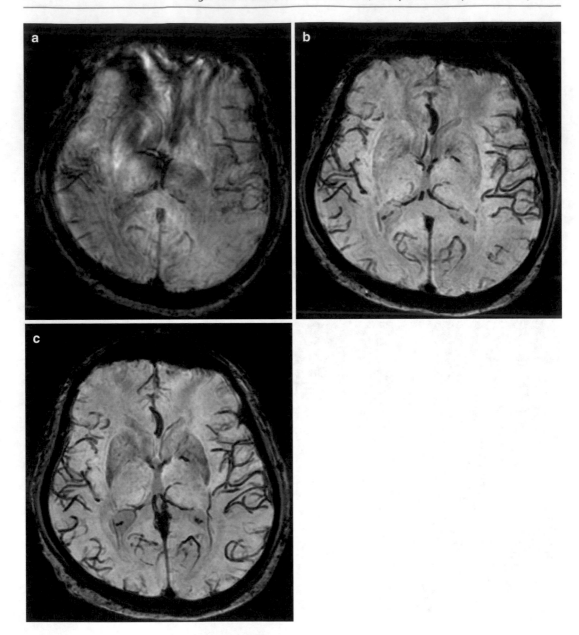

Fig. 1.5 Axial SWI, January 2019 (**a**), February (**b**), May (**c**). Putamen and globus pallidus did not reveal abnormal signal intensity on both sides, in May those structures were hypointense

and tremor significantly improved in combination with physical therapy.

The latest brain MRI was performed in October 2019 and did not reveal changes in comparison to MRI performed in May.

1.1   Voltage-Gated Potassium Channel (VGKC)-Complex Antibody Limbic Encephalitis

Autoimmune limbic encephalitis (AILE) is one of the most common causes of non-infectious encephalitis presenting an immune response against neuronal autoantigen with the production of antibodies. Anti-neuronal antibodies are divided into three groups.

In paraneoplastic AILE, antibodies are against paraneoplastic intraneuronal antigens (INAab). Intracellular antibodies, also known as onconeural antibodies, are the result of an underlying tumour. INA antibodies (e.g. anti-Hu, anti-Yo, anti-Ta) are most likely not directly pathogenic and probably an epiphenomenon of T-cell-mediated immune response. They are not directly pathogenic and can be very useful as a marker of disease. Because of cytotoxic neuronal damage, these patients often do not respond well to immunotherapy, and their symptoms are mostly irreversible [1, 2].

In non-neoplastic AILE, antibodies are against cell surface antigens (CSAab) or against synaptic antigens (SyAab). The CSAab (e.g. anti-NMDARab, VGKCab, VGCCab) target molecules involved in neurotransmission leading to neuronal dysfunction. They may have agonistic or antagonistic effects on the receptors, block ion channel pores or disrupt the interaction with neighbouring molecules. They could also alter receptor localization at the membrane or cause receptor internalization, thus reducing cell surface expression of receptors [3]. The SyAab are believed to contribute to the alteration of neurotransmitter release. Patients with AIE associated with CSAab have a more favourable prognosis due to reversible neurological symptoms and good response to immune suppressive

therapy. Although these antibodies are predominately considered non-paraneoplastic, in up to 30% of cases, an underlying tumour has been identified, most commonly SCLC or thymoma.

The voltage-gated potassium channel (VGKC) complex is a transmembrane potassium channel that establishes resting membrane potential and generates neuronal action potentials, therefore adjusts the neuronal excitability of central and peripheral nervous system. It was previously thought that autoantibodies target the VGKC complex itself, but according to different studies in the past few years, those antibodies actually are directed against secreted cell surface proteins associated with the complex: leucine-rich glioma inactivated 1(LGI1) and less frequently contactin-associated protein-2 (CASPR2) [2, 4].

LGI1 is a neuronal secreted protein released by presynaptic membrane that interacts with presynaptic ADAM23 and postsynaptic ADAM22 to affect the signal transduction between the synapses by the VGKCs and postsynaptic membrane α-amino-3-hydroxy-5-methyl-4-isoxazole propionate receptors (AMPAR). This combination is necessary for the inhibition of signal conduction. LGI1 antibody reduces the interaction of LGI1–ADAM and aggregation of AMPAR (reversibly) [2, 5]. Patients with anti-LGI1 antibodies are typically men older than 40 years who presents with limbic encephalitis characterized by subacute memory disturbances accompanied by various neuropsychiatric symptoms, behavioural abnormalities, faciobrachial dystonic seizures, hyponatremia and epileptic seizures. Some scientists think that hyponatraemia in autoimmune encephalitis related to LGI1 antibody may be caused by improper secretion syndrome of antidiuretic hormone, and it might be related to the simultaneous LGI1 expressions of the hypothalamus and kidney.

CASPR2 is an axonal transmembrane protein of the neurexin superfamily that binds to contactin-2. It is involved in clustering of potassium channels in myelinated axons. CASPR2 is also present in the hippocampus and cerebellum. Anti-CASPR2 antibodies are associated with encephalitis, peripheral nerve hyperexcitability (also known as acquired neuromyotonia or Isaacs syndrome) or a combination of both (Morvan syndrome, characterized by encephalopathy with prominent psychiatric symptoms, insomnia, dysautonomia and neuromyotonia and almost exclusively affects male patients). Patients are often men about 60 years old, although it has been described in patients aged 19–80 years [1, 3].

About half of patients with anti-VGKC encephalitis do not present antibodies against LGI1 or CASPR2. These specific groups of patients develop a wide variety of clinical syndromes. It is also a heterogeneous group of clinical syndromes linked to these VGKC antibodies in which LGI1 and CASPR2 antibodies are not present. This wide range of syndromes includes not only diseases restricted to the central nervous system, but could affect the peripheral nervous system (neuropathy, neuropathic pain) [6, 7]. The precise antigens are unknown in all these cases: it is not even clear whether they are intracellular or extracellular. Furthermore, responses to immunosuppressive treatment in the cases described above vary greatly, which highlights the relevance of the diagnostic value and pathogenesis of these antibodies [7, 8].

Definite diagnosis of AILE is based on a clinical history suggestive of AILE, detection of antibodies in the CSF and/or serum, MRI findings, functional imaging with positron emission tomography and electroencephalography.

Brain MRI in AILE with VGKC-associated antibodies reveals unilateral or bilateral hippocampal and amygdala involvement often accompanied by basal ganglia involvement. Involved structures are enlarged and hyperintense on T2WI and FLAIR sequences. Diffusion restriction in the T2 hyperintense areas with contrast enhancement is visible in up to 30–40% cases. Patients with restricted diffusion and contrast enhancement of involved structures are at increased risk of developing post-inflammatory atrophy that contributes to persistent memory impairment and the neurological disability seen in patients in due course of the disease [1, 6, 8, 9]. On follow-up investigations, swelling of involved structures is followed by atrophy, while hyperintensity persists in most patients in different extent.

FDG–PET imaging usually reveals hypermetabolism in the involved structures, as well as hypometabolism in rare cases. It significantly increases the sensitivity for abnormalities in limbic encephalitis revealing altered glucose metabolism even in normally appearing temporal lobe structures on MRI [1]. Additionally, FDG–PET more often shows extralimbic abnormalities (mainly hypermetabolism), e.g. in the brainstem, cerebellum or cerebral cortex, and seems to correlate more closely with clinical symptoms than MRI [1].

Results from routine CSF tests are usually normal, although patients may present moderate pleocytosis and increased protein levels.

If AILE is suspected, routine serum tests for autoimmune encephalitis antibodies are the first performed because blood is more sensitive than CSF. The positive rate of specific antibody detection in CSF is lower than that in serum: even if CSF is positive for specific antibodies, its titre is only 1–10% of a serum titre. Both serum and CSF antibody titres can decrease or increase with the disease remission and relapse, respectively.

The diagnosis of LGI1 antibody encephalitis need to be distinguished from viral encephalitis, Hashimoto's encephalopathy, Creutzfeldt–Jakob disease (CJD) and other forms of autoimmune encephalitis. In combination with clinical manifestations, laboratory tests and imaging examinations, the diagnosis of LGI1 antibody encephalitis is usually correct; however, it should be noted that increased LGI1 antibody titres were also found in a pathologically confirmed CJD case [10].

First-line therapies for the disease include intravenous glucocorticoid therapy and immunoglobulin and plasma exchange, with early combinatorial treatments providing better efficacy. In addition to these combinatorial treatments, it is sometimes necessary to supplement treatment with cyclophosphamide or rituximab.

It is not easy to make diagnosis of autoimmune limbic encephalitis. Due to clinical symptoms and acute or subacute onset, those patients are mistaken for psychiatric cases in number of cases. It was almost the case with our patient: his leading symptoms on the admission were neurological symptoms, but was actually admitted due to electrolyte disorder. Headache and vertigo could have been symptoms in course of influenza. Electrolyte disorder was presumed to be a result of vomiting and diuretic therapy, and psychiatric and neurological symptoms were mistaken for organic mental disorders in course of his former alcohol addiction (underwent alcohol addiction treatment 4 years before the disease onset) and vitamin B_{12} hypovitaminosis. Neither general radiologist nor neuroradiologist was informed of his clinical condition and course of his symptoms, only information both had was clinician referral of central pontine myelinolysis and hyponatraemia. Both MRIs performed in January and February 2019 did not reveal changes specific for central pontine myelinolysis, but with little information radiologists had, possible differential were extrapontine myelinolysis or possible lymbic encephalitis. In extrapontine myelinolysis basal ganglia, ventrolateral thalamus, internal, external and extreme capsule and splenium of corpus callosum are typically involved [11]. Temporal lobes are not involved, although cases of extrapontine myelinolysis with amygdala involvement have been reported in the literature.

Since tumour markers, chest and abdominal CTs were negative for neoplasm, we had to wait for the results of serum and CSF CSAab and INAab because one of consulted neurologists suspected AILE may be in question. All tested antibodies, as well as LGI1Ab and CASPR2Ab were negative in serum and CSF except slightly elevated anti-VGKC Ab in serum. Attending neurologist, who was the last to examine patient during hospitalisation, did not consider definitely AILE, but ordered control MRI and most of the specific antigens in serum in 2 months. In May 2019, patient neurological symptoms progressed as well as the level of serum anti-VGKCAb. Therefore, diagnosis of the anti-VGKCAb AILE

(LGI1 and CASPR2 negative) was finally made and the treatment started. As already presented, pulse corticosteroid therapy and later on intravenous immunoglobulin treatment were only partially successful. Very good results were finally achieved with monoclonal antibody treatment, which is consistent with the fact that in case of anti-VGKCAb AILE, LGI1 and CAPSR2 negative, response to immunosuppressive treatment varies greatly. Our patient did not have epileptic seizures as a symptom during the course of his disease. He was without seizures on follow-ups, although hippocampal and amygdala volume reduction have been described on follow-up MRI.

Not only in this chapter, but in several chapters to follow, I will try to emphasize the problem most of us is facing, which is, as you can anticipate, a lack of proper and complete information of patient condition, course of disease, laboratory and other findings, patient social and epidemiological history when asked from clinicians. Clinician referral in the case, central pontine myelinolysis and hyponatremia were not sufficient as referral information for MRI.

References

1. Guerin J, et al. Autoimmune epilepsy: findings on MRI and FDG-PET. Br J Radiol. 2019;92:20170869.
2. Van Coevorden-Hameete MH, et al. Molecular and cellular mechanisms underlying anti-neuronal antibody mediated disorders of the central nervous system. Autoimmun Rev. 2014;13:299–312.
3. Dutra LA, et al. Autoimmune encephalitis: a review of diagnosis and treatment. Arq Neuropsiquiatr. 2017;76(1):41–9.
4. Langille MM, Desai J. Encephalitis due to antibodies to voltage gated potassium channel (VGKC) with cerebellar involvement in a teenager. Ann Indian Acad Neur. 2015;18(2):238–9.
5. Wang M, et al. Clinical features of limbic encephalitis with LGI I antibody. Neuropsychiatr Dis Treat. 2017;13:1589–96.
6. Hacohen Y, et al. A clinico-radiological phenotype of voltage-gated potassium channel complex antibody-mediated disorder presenting with seizures and basal ganglia changes. Dev Med Child Neurol. 2012;54(12):1157–9.

7. Agarwal KA, et al. Autoimmune limbic encephalitis in a patient with acute encephalopathy and hyponatremia. Case Rep Med. 2019;2019:9051738.
8. Montojo MT, et al. Clinical spectrum and diagnostic value of antibodies against the potassium channel-related protein complex. Neurologia. 2015;30(5):295–301.
9. Heine J, et al. Imaging of autoimmune encephalitis – relevance for clinical practice and hippocampal function. Neuroscience. 2015;309:68–83.
10. Celicanin M, et al. Autoimmune encephalitis associated with voltage-gated potassium channels-complex and leucine-rich glioma-inactivated 1 antibodies – a national cohort study. Eur J Neurol. 2017;0:1–7.
11. Bhatia S, et al. Cerebral encephalopathy with extrapontine myelinolysis in a case of postpartum hypernatremia. Indian J Radiol Imag. 2014;24(1):57–60.

Cranial Bone Changes in Megaloblastic Anaemia Due to Anorexia Nervosa

In April 2017, a 28-year-old female patient was hospitalized due to a vitamin deficiency and protein-energy malnutrition due to anorexia nervosa (AN). The patient had university degree, lived alone and did not have a partner, and relations with parents were disturbed. She claimed she was teased in high school about her weight, although she weighed not more than 65 kg at the time. She suffered from eating disorder for the past 10 years during which she was not in psychiatrist treatment although she was referred by general practitioner for a consultation. Her opinion was her ideal body weight would be 35 kg; she was eating only salt sticks, apples and yogurt.

On admission, she was anorexic, weighed 44.5 kg (163 cm tall), had headache and vertigo, abdominal pain and cramps and peripheral oedema. Laboratory findings revealed megaloblastic macrocytic anaemia, leukopenia and thrombocytopenia, heavy hypoalbuminaemia, low serum levels of glucose, creatinine, chloride and calcium. Aspartate transaminase, lactate dehydrogenase and alkaline phosphatase levels were low.

Vitamin B_{12} serum level was normal, and folate serum level was low, as well as copper and ceruloplasmin. Sodium and potassium levels, inorganic phosphates and total magnesium were normal.

During hospitalization, she was in endocrinologist treatment, while psychiatrist, neurologist and nutritionist were consulted.

Bone marrow puncture confirmed megaloblastic anaemia. Abdominal ultrasound revealed moderate amount of free fluid in the upper abdomen—together with peripheral oedema, it was a result of hypoalbuminaemia.

Neurologist was consulted due to headaches and vertigo, and brain MRI was recommended: it revealed bone changes that could be attributable to megaloblastic anaemia (Fig. 2.1).

According to attending psychiatrist, at first she expressed the desire for proper psychiatric treatment, but before she was discharged from the hospital, she was not eager to give it a try anymore: she was afraid of getting weight.

The patient was admitted to our hospital again in December 2019 because her life was seriously endangered by the AN. Between April 2017 and December 2019, she visited the psychiatrist from time to time, without continuous, proper psychiatric treatment because she was refusing to take medication and food. All the mentioned laboratory findings from 2017 were the same or worse. Dual-energy X-ray absorptiometry (DXA) revealed decreased mineral bone density (MBD). Psychiatrist, neurologist, haematologist, gastroenterologist and nutritionist were consulted again.

According to attending psychiatrist, she was not cooperating in treatment, she was stubborn and firm in sticking to habits that endangered her life: refused food, drinking only half a litre of water and a glass of chamomile tea without sugar

M. Špero, H. Vavro, *Neuroradiology - Images vs Symptoms*,
https://doi.org/10.1007/978-3-030-69213-1_2

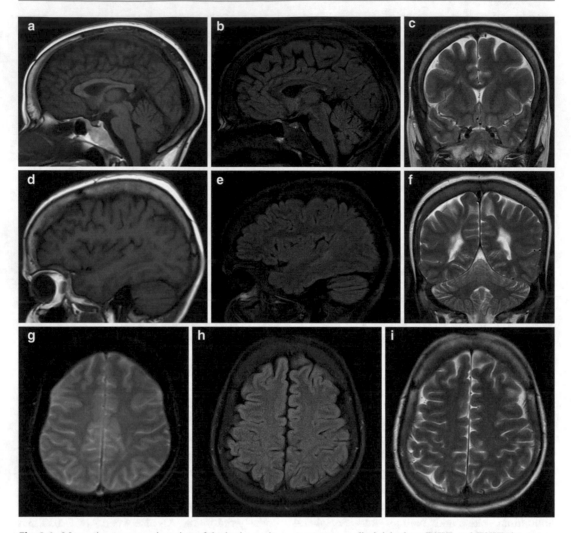

Fig. 2.1 Magnetic resonance imaging of the brain, sagittal T1WI (**a**, **d**), FLAIR (**b**, **e**), coronal T2WI (**c**, **f**), axial T2*WI (**g**), FLAIR (**h**), T2WI (**i**) revealed thickened clivus, frontal and parietal bones—frontal bone was more thickened than parietal bones. Signal intensity of the bone marrow was diminished on T1WI and T2WI due to reconverted bone marrow in long-term megaloblastic anaemia due to folate deficiency in AN. T1W signal of the subcutaneous tissue was normal

or honey per day. She also revealed affective dullness and delusional beliefs regarding diet, body weight and self-image.

The patient also refused transfusion of red cell concentrates, vitamin supplements, parenteral nutrition and a nutrition diet plan. She was obviously a person who lacked capacity to make proper decision regarding specific treatment in a psychiatric institution providing specialized for the treatment of eating disorder.

The patient was discharged from the hospital at her own request, while a centre for social welfare was informed about the necessity to start the process of capacity evaluation or appointment of guardian, so a specific and needed treatment could begin.

2.1 Cranial Bone Changes in Megaloblastic Anaemia Due to Anorexia Nervosa

Anorexia nervosa is an eating disorder characterized by an irrational fear of food as well as extreme, life-threatening weight loss. It is classified as a mental illness starting most often during a person's teenage years or young adulthood, women are ten times likely to be diagnosed compared to men. Patients who suffer from AN have a distorted body image and an excessive, obsessive fear of obesity, even when they are significantly underweight: they do not necessarily lose their appetite but rather obsessively control and restrict their food intake. One in five patients with AN dies due to complications of the disease.

Megaloblastic anaemia is macrocytic anaemia resulting most often from deficiencies of vitamin B_{12} and folate. Megaloblasts are large nucleated red blood cell precursors with non-condensed chromatin due to impaired DNA synthesis: mean corpuscular volume is >100 fL [1, 2]. Anaemia is undoubtedly a common and multifactorial complication of AN. In most cases, it is a moderate, transitory and asymptomatic anaemia eventually corrected by itself with appropriate and progressive refeeding. Anaemia due to folate and/or vitamin B_{12} deprivation is rare within AN patients but has also been reported. It can be associated with a slight leukopenia, while thrombocytopenia occurs in case of folate deficiency [2, 3]. Vitamin B_{12} and folate therapy has been proven effective.

Among the many adverse physical sequelae of AN, bone health is impacted by starvation and can be permanently impaired over the course of the illness. Magnetic resonance imaging is the best imaging modality for evaluating bone marrow because it provides good resolution and clearly distinguishes fat from other tissues. Normal yellow (inactive, fatty) bone marrow appears hyperintense on T1W images due to its high fat content. Normal red (active, hematopoietic) bone marrow is hypointense compared to yellow marrow on T1W images [4, 5].

The bone marrow of neonates is predominantly red, and hematopoietic cells are replaced by fatty tissue with aging. Conversion of marrow from the red to the yellow form begins in the peripheral skeleton and progresses centrally. In healthy subjects, red marrow is almost completely converted to yellow marrow during the first and second decades of life. Marrow re-conversion is the reverse process; it begins in the axial skeleton and proceeds to the appendicular skeleton. Re-conversion occurs under stressful conditions such as anaemia and infiltrative marrow disorders, when the demand for blood cell production exceeds the existing marrow's ability to manufacture these products. The extent of re-conversion depends on the severity and duration of the stimulus [4, 5].

In chronic anaemia, re-converted bone marrow (CBM) appears as diffuse or focal areas of diminished signal intensity on T1W images and exhibits a variable appearance on T2W images [5]. CBM is thickened in long time haemolytic anaemia, and to lesser degree, in non-haemolytic anaemia. Our patient is an example of untreated AN during which she has endangered her own life. She had macrocytic megaloblastic anaemia due to folate deficiency and thrombocytopenia as well. Brain MRI was performed due to headache and vertigo and revealed thickened cranial bones and its signal intensity changes due to re-converted CBM) in a process of long-term megaloblastic anaemia (Fig. 2.1). There was no sign of a brain volume deficit with increased cerebrospinal fluid, but she had changes typical for periventricular leukomalacia (PVL) related to white matter injury of prematurity (Figs. 2.1f and 2.2). PVL is related to the selective maturation-dependent vulnerability of cells of oligodendrocyte lineage to changes of hypoxia-ischaemia.

Neuroimaging techniques have been useful tools for accurate investigation of brain structure and function in eating disorders, mainly in AN. In general, CT and MRI studies of AN have reported brain volume deficits and increased cerebrospinal fluid including reduction in total grey and white matter, sulcal widening and ventricular enlargement, reduction in cerebral gyri in size, indicating the effects of starvation in the brain [6, 7]. It appears that the grey and white matter increase significantly following weight restoration. Some of these findings suggest that changes are most likely to be due to neuronal damage secondary to malnutrition, with possible regeneration of myelin accounting for the general reversibility [6, 7].

With progressive reductions in body weight, normal hyperintense T1W signal is lost from the subcutaneous fat and the orbits as well [7]. These signal intensity changes are also seen at CT as an increase in attenuation, and they may reverse with weight restoration.

Regarding the patient, brain MRI did not show diminished T1W signal of the subcutaneous and orbital fat, but revealed mild parotid glands enlargement due to sialosis. Parotid gland sialosis

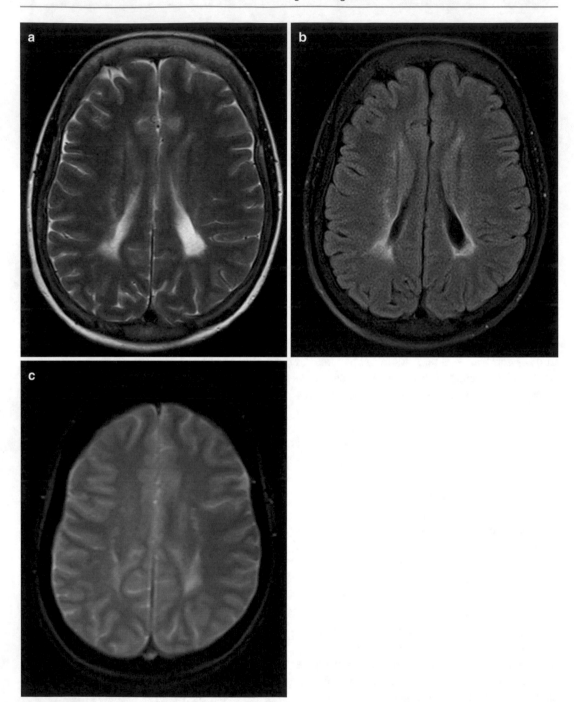

Fig. 2.2 Brain magnetic resonance imaging, axial T2WI (**a**), FLAIR (**b**) and T2*WI (**c**) revealed end-stage of periventricular leukomalacia: increased signal intensity in frontal and bilateral parietal periventricular white matter due to gliosis (**a**, **b**). Enlargement of the atria of the lateral ventricles with a decrease in volume of the adjacent white matter, walls of the lateral ventricles have a slightly wavy appearance (**a**, **b**). No evidence of chronic haemorrhage (**c**)

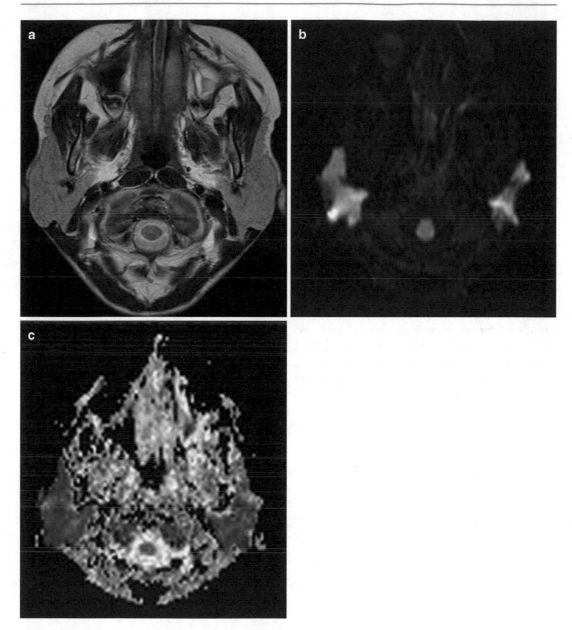

Fig. 2.3 Parotid gland sialosis in anorexia nervosa. MRI axial T2WI (**a**), DWI (**b**) and ADC (**c**) revealed mild bilateral enlargement of parotid glands, slightly hyperintense on T2WI (**a**) with decreased diffusion (**b**, **c**) possible due to cellular enlargement and gland swelling

is non-inflammatory, non-neoplastic, painless enlargement of the gland associated with a variety of conditions including alcoholism, endocrine disorders and malnutrition which in our society usually results from AN. It is recurrent and usually bilateral, caused by hypertrophy of the acinar component [8, 9]. Cellular enlargement leads to parotid gland hypertrophy and swelling (Fig. 2.3), which may be detectable at CT or MR imaging [9]. CT features include increased attenuation of the gland at unenhanced CT due to loss of the normal hypoattenuating intraparotid fat, while MRI features include slight decrease in T1W signal due to lower fat content and slight increase in T2W signal (Fig. 2.3a). Fatty replacement and reduction in size are features of sialosis in late stages [9].

The patient had hypothalamic amenorrhea and decreased MBD as well. Hypothalamic amenorrhea is a hallmark of AN and is potentially reversible with weight restoration. Return of menstrual cycle is expected as a sign of improved physiologic function during AN recovery [10]. Decreased MBD is common consequence of a restrictive eating disorder such as AN. The body draws on its nutrient-rich skeletal reserve to support physiologic function in the absence of adequate oral intake. Over time, this process leads to decreased MBD. Among adult women with AN, those who developed the disease as adolescents have lower bone density measures than those who developed the disease later in life, supporting the critical relationship between adolescent nutritional intake, peak bone mass accrual and life-long bone health [10]. Although skeletal losses that occur during the course of AN can improve with recovery, full recovery cannot always be expected.

References

1. Mamou G, et al. Anemia in anorexia nervosa: the best way to deal with it – an overview of literature. J Hum Nutr Food Sci. 2016;4(1):1081–8.
2. Nagao T, Hirokawa M. Diagnosis and treatment of macrocytic anemias in adults. J Gen Fam Med. 2017;18(5):200–4.
3. Filippo D, et al. Hematological complications in anorexia nervosa. Eur J Clin Nutr. 2016;70:1305–8.
4. Shah G, et al. Incidence and evaluation of incidental abnormal bone marrow signal on magnetic resonance imaging. Sci World J. 2014;2014:380814.
5. Yildirim T, et al. MRI evaluation of cranial bone marrow signal intensity and thickness in chronic anemia. Eur J Radiol. 2005;53:125–30.
6. Jauregui-Lobera I. Neuroimaging in eating disorders. Neuropsychiatr Dis Treat. 2011;7:577–84.
7. Bowden DJ, et al. Radiology of eating disorders: a pictorial review. Radiographics. 2013;33:1171–93.
8. Jagtap SV, et al. Sialosis: cytomorphological significance in the diagnosis of uncommon entity. J Cytol. 2017;34(1):51–2.
9. Ugga L, et al. Diagnostic work-up in obstructive and inflammatory salivary gland disorder. Acta Otorhinolaryngol Ital. 2017;37(2):83–93.
10. Donaldson AA, Gordon CM. Skeletal complications of eating disorders. Metabolism. 2015;64(9):943–51.

Multinodular and Vacuolating Neuronal Tumour (MVNT)

At the beginning of summer 2019, a woman in her early 50s was admitted to hospital on account of severe dizziness with nausea and left ear tinnitus. The vertigo had started that morning, while left tinnitus had already been bothering her for a month. Apart from not being able to stand up due to dizziness, there were no other neurological symptoms. Colour Doppler study of the carotid and vertebral arteries was normal. Cardiovascular and ophthalmic exams revealed no abnormalities.

Brain CT exam done on admission did not demonstrate any posterior fossa nor temporal bone lesions (Fig. 3.1).

As the symptoms were persistent, an MRI examination of the brain was called for (Fig. 3.2). The MRI did not reveal the cause of dizziness and vertigo, but did yield some more information on the right-sided frontal lesion.

On account of morphology, location and signals, a diagnosis of a multinodular and vacuolating neuronal tumour was proposed as most likely.

EEG was within normal limits. The frontal lesion was felt to be an incidental finding, so the neurosurgeon was not inclined to invasive methods of workup—the proposal was to do a follow-up MRI in 4 months.

The symptomatic vertigo therapy has eventually yielded results, and the patient was discharged from the hospital, with instructions to come back for a MRI scan in 4 months (Fig. 3.3).

3.1 Multinodular and Vacuolating Neuronal Tumour (MVNT)

MVNT has been recognized as an entity in 2016, by the latest revision of World Health Organization Classification of Tumours of the Central Nervous System. It appears to be a unique cytoarchitectural pattern of a gangliocytoma; the tumour cells demonstrate glial and/or neuronal differentiation. MVNT is low-grade, made of multiple nodules with vacuolation and may be malformative (dysplastic) rather than neoplastic [1].

Histopathological findings feature neurocpithelial cells with stromal vacuolation arranged in nodules sited in the deep cortical layer and superficial subcortical white matter, oriented perpendicular to the cortex. There is essentially no mitotic activity [2]. This correlates with MR imaging appearance—a cluster of variably sized nodular lesions in the superficial white matter, lower in cellularity compared to the adjacent white matter.

MVNTs are negative for KIAA1549–BRAF gene fusions related to microvascular proliferation in gliomas. They also do not demonstrate mutations involving IDH1 or IDH2, ATRX, TP53, TERT, CIC, FUBP1, PRKCA, CDKN2A and FGFR1. However, they have been proved to harbour MAP 2K1 exon 2 mutations, non-V600E BRAF mutations and FGFR2 fusions. On account

M. Špero, H. Vavro, *Neuroradiology - Images vs Symptoms*, https://doi.org/10.1007/978-3-030-69213-1_3

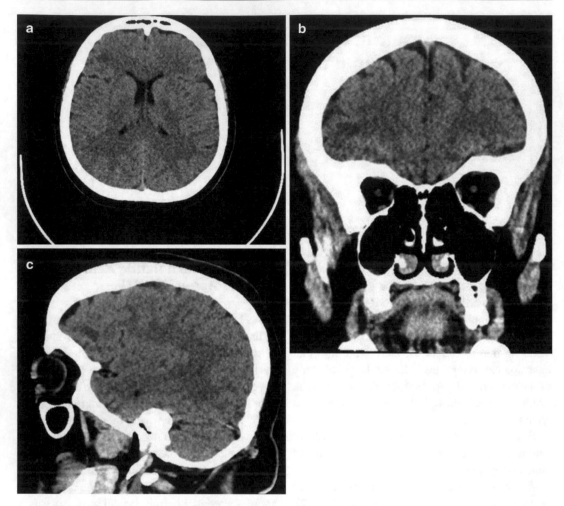

Fig. 3.1 Axial (**a**), coronal (**b**) and sagittal (**c**) reformats of a brain CT scan showing a small hypodense area in the right-sided frontal lobe which was reported as a "chronic ischaemic lesion"

of these findings, it has been proposed that they should be placed within the "Neuronal and mixed neuronal-glial tumours" section as a distinctive WHO grade I tumour [3]. These latest findings of clonal genetic alterations harboured by MVNTs favour a neoplastic over a dysplastic origin.

Although it has been considered an epilepsy-related tumour, MVNT is often clinically silent and found incidentally, like in this case. Most patients present with non-specific, non-focal

symptoms. Some of them present with seizure disorders but even then a strong clinical and imaging correlation has to be established because epileptic foci may not be related to a MVNT found on MRI [4, 5]. It appears to be an indolent benign lesion which should most often be left alone and merely followed by MRI imaging on a regular basis. Patient age in studies ranged from late teens to late 70s, with a mean age in early 40s. While in one retrospective study [6] the most

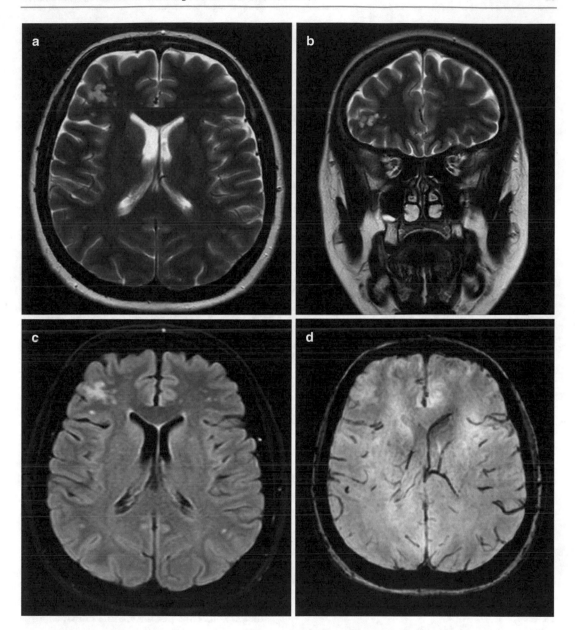

Fig. 3.2 Axial and coronal T2WI (**a**, **b**), axial T2-FLAIR FS (**c**), SWI (**d**) and ADC map (**e**) and axial post-contrast T1WI (**f**) demonstrate a cluster of non-enhancing subcortical nodular lesions, hyperintense in T2WI and hypoin-tense in T1WI, with ever so slightly increased diffusion, without evidence of haemorrhage. No mass effect nor perifocal oedema. Again, no posterior fossa lesions were seen

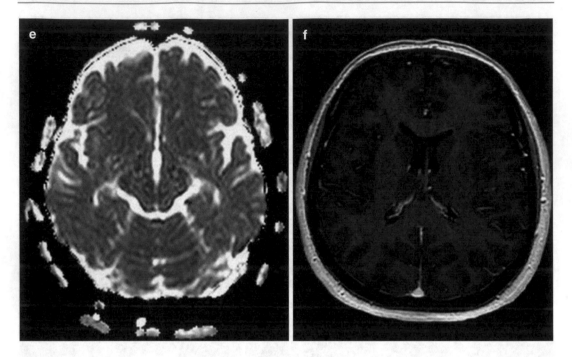

Fig. 3.2 (continued)

tumours were found in frontal and parietal lobes, in another literature review, there was a strong affinity for temporal lobes. Superficial subcortical white matter location was common to all cases in both papers, but there are sporadic cases of deep parenchymal involvement [3]. During 2–4 years of follow-up, intracranial status in both operated and non-operated patients remained stable, without recurring lesions in surgical patients and with no change in size and signal in other patients who did not undergo surgery for MVNT.

Conventional MRI is the mainstay of imaging for the diagnosis of MVNT, with specific imaging features: coalescent juxtacortical non-enhancing nodules ("bubbly" appearance) which are hyperintense in T2WI (including FLAIR) and slightly hypointense in T1WI. There is no visible cortical involvement nor mass-effect. Increased diffusivity is compatible with low tumour cellularity and lack of mitotic activity. On MR spectroscopy, there is a relative increase in choline/creatine and choline/NAA peak ratio, while perfusion imaging does not demonstrate significant

change in CBV values compared to normal brain tissue.

The main differential diagnoses include:

- DNET, which unlike MVNT typically exhibits a cortical location, demonstrates partial suppression of T2 signal in FLAIR sequence (with a hyperintense rim) and may enhance with gadolinium contrast.
- Focal cortical dysplasia, which features cortical thickening and blurring of the grey–white matter interface, possibly with abnormal cortical gyration.
- Enlarged Virchow–Robin perivascular spaces, which follow CSF signal intensity in all sequences (attenuated in FLAIR) and have a predilection for the mesencephalic area.

Therapy for MVNT is in most cases unnecessary as they are clinically silent, incidental lesions. Surgical therapy is indicated only if there is a strong correlation between MVNT location and patient's symptoms (e.g. intractable seizures).

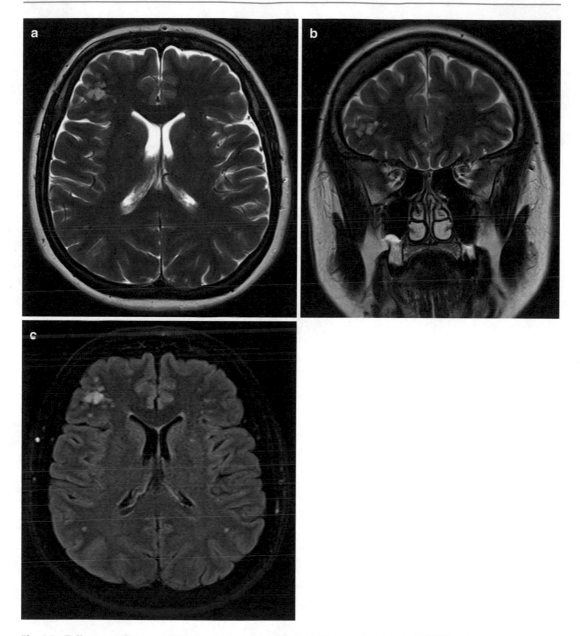

Fig. 3.3 Follow-up MRI exam of the brain, 4 months after the initial examination. Axial T2WI (**a**), coronal T2WI (**b**) and axial T2-FLAIR image (**c**) show no interval change in signal and size of the MVNT

References

1. Louis DN, et al. The 2016 World Health Organization classification of tumors of the central nervous system: a summary. Acta Neuropathol. 2016;131(6):803–20. https://doi.org/10.1007/s00401-016-1545-1.
2. Narvaez EO, et al. Multinodular and vacuolating neuronal tumor in the brain depth - atypical presentation of a new tumor: a case report. J Mol Genet Med. 2020;14:453. https://doi.org/10.37421/jmgm.2020.14.453.
3. Kodama S, et al. Multinodular and vacuolating neuronal tumor (MVNT): a presumably incidental and asymptomatic case in an intractable epilepsy patient. Clin Neurophysiol Pract. 2019;4:164–7. https://doi.org/10.1016/j.cnp.2019.05.003.
4. Makrakis D, et al. Multinodular and vacuolating neuronal tumor incidentally discovered in a young man: conventional and advanced MRI features. Radiol Case

Rep. 2018;13(5):960–4. https://doi.org/10.1016/j.radcr.2018.07.016.

5. Buffa GB, et al. Multinodular and vacuolating neuronal tumor of the cerebrum (MVNT): a case series and review of the literature. J Neuroradiol. 2020;47(3):216–20. https://doi.org/10.1016/j.neurad.2019.05.010.

6. Shitara S, et al. Multinodular and vacuolating neuronal tumor: a case report and literature review. Surg Neurol Int. 2018;9:63. https://doi.org/10.4103/sni.sni_348_17.

Intracranial Extra-Axial Teratoma in an Adult Female Patient

A female patient, 37 years old, came to our department for the brain CT as an outpatient. CT was recommended by a general practitioner due to headaches lasting for a few months. Headaches were intermittent, described as a squeezing pain around the head.

Expansile extra-axial neoplasm was reported on CT, possible degenerated and calcified meningioma due to attenuation coefficients of the lesion and calcifications (Fig. 4.1). The patient was scheduled for the brain MRI (Fig. 4.2): after MRI, she was admitted to the hospital for neurosurgery.

After brain MRI, it was obvious that the neoplasm was not a degenerated calcified meningioma. The patient underwent a right-sided parasagittal frontoparietal craniotomy: mostly calcified mass with several central soft areas was completely removed. Tumour was invading and destroying a large part of the cerebral falx. According to intraoperative pathologist consultation, tumour tissue was mature cartilage tissue. After a few days, final pathologist report was mature teratoma: tumour consisted of mature cartilage tissue, several fragments of bone tissue and mature fat tissue (Fig. 4.3).

Follow-up brain MRI performed 3 months after the operation did not reveal tumour recurrence; the patient was without headaches and any neurological deficits.

4.1 Intracranial Extra-Axial Teratoma in an Adult Female Patient

Teratomas belong to the class of germ cell tumours (GCTs) and originate from totipotent germ cells.

Germ cell tumours are neoplasms of germinal origin occurring in the gonads and extra-gonadal sites. Those tumours are uncommon primary neoplasms of the central nervous system (CNS) and comprise 3–11% of all intracranial neoplasms in children and 1% of all primary intracranial neoplasms in adults [1]. According to the 2016 World Health Organization guidelines, CNS germ cell tumours are classified into germinomas and non-germinomatous germ cell tumours including embryonal carcinomas, yolk sac tumours, choriocarcinomas, teratomas, teratomas with malignant transformation, and mixed germ cell tumours. Teratomas are further classified into mature and immature teratomas [2].

Mature teratomas (MTs) are a type of GCTs containing well-differentiated tissue elements of each of the three germ cell layers: endoderm, mesoderm and ectoderm. Immature teratoma consists of components resembling foetal tissue, whereas teratomas with malignant transformation are extremely rare and are characterized with additional malignant somatic tissue [3].

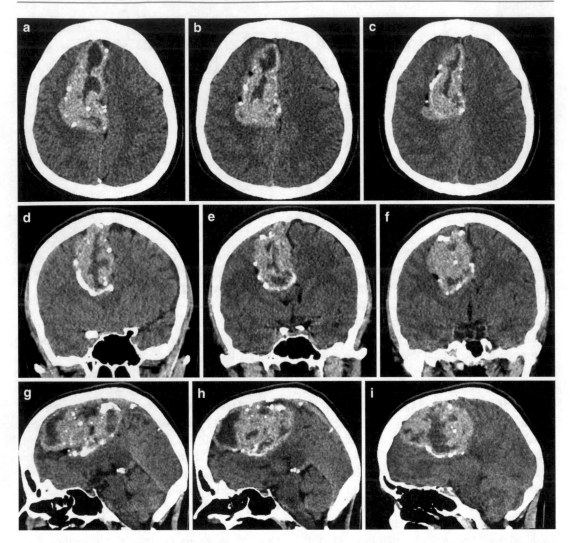

Fig. 4.1 Computed tomography of the brain (non-contrast), axial (**a–c**), coronal (**d–f**), sagittal (**g–i**) scans, revealed supratentorial large right parasagittal, dural-based frontal extra-axial mass: lobulated, well-circumscribed, heterogeneous, mainly hyperdense with irregular hypodense areas, irregular calcifications and a few very small, oval hypodensities at the lateral edge of the mass mistaken for a CSF between the mass and surrounding brain parenchyma. It compressed adjacent gyrus cinguli, ventral part of the corpus callosum body and frontal part of the right lateral ventricle. Tumour did not show cystic component. There was no oedema in surrounding brain parenchyma

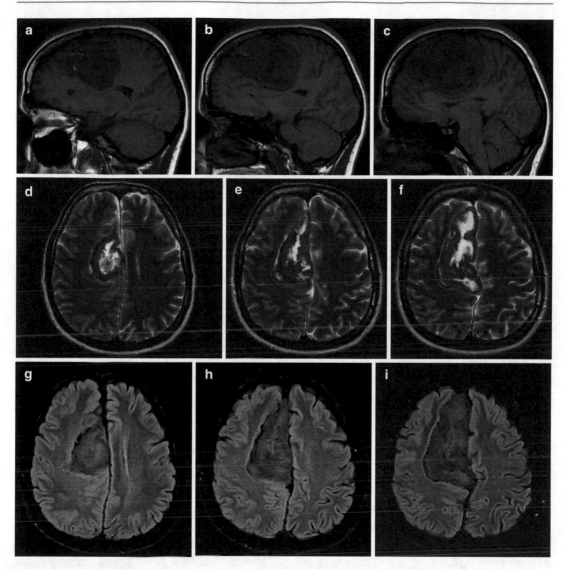

Fig. 4.2 Brain magnetic resonance imaging, sagittal T1WI (**a–c**), axial T2WI (**d–f**), FLAIR FS (**g–i**), DWI (**j**), ADC (**k**), SWI (**l**), post-contrast T1WI (**m–o**). Large right frontal and parasagittal, cerebral falx-based extra-axial mass was reported as well-circumscribed, heterogeneous signal intensity, iso- to low signal intensity on T1WI, hypointense on T2WI and FLAIR FS with hyperintense inhomogeneous areas on T2WI. There was no restricted diffusion (**j**, **k**) or haemorrhage (**l**). A few small, oval hypodensities at the lateral edge of the mass mistaken for a CSF on CT were hyperintense on T1WI due to fat. After intravenous administration of gadolinium contrast media, there was only linear rim contrast enhancement. Cerebral falx showed mild reactive contrast enhancement. There was no oedema in surrounding brain parenchyma, the mass did not compress or invade superior sagittal sinus

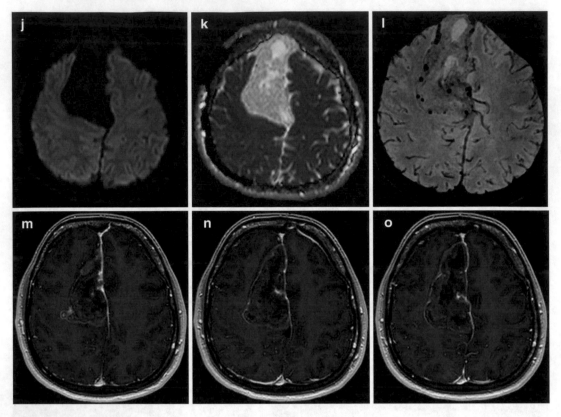

Fig. 4.2 (continued)

Intracranial MTs are tumours with a very low incidence (0.2%) and male predominance (5:1). The prevalence is much higher in the earlier decades of life, with one peak in the neonatal and infancy period and another peak in children ages of 5–14 years [4, 5].

According to the embryonic theory, GCTs arise from a mis-migrational pluripotent germ cell. It is proposed that germinomas arise from germ cells, while other non-germinomatous GCTs, including teratomas, occur due to mis-folding or misplacement of embryonic cells into the lateral mesoderm, causing their entrapment in various parts of the CNS [5, 6].

Clinical symptoms depend on the location of the tumour: MTs remain asymptomatic until they become sufficiently large to produce a mass effect or obstructive hydrocephalus.

The imaging characteristics of MTs depend on the cellular components and their products. Those usually have cystic and solid component. MTs often display heterogeneous densities on CT imaging and heterogeneous signal intensities on MR images reflecting various components contained within the lesion, such as soft tissue, cartilage, bone, fatty tissue and calcification. Therefore, various MRI signal intensities are reported in the literature, which range from heterogeneous hyperintense on T1WI, hypointense on T2WI, to lesions that are hypointense on T1WI and hyperintense on T2W images. Diffusion could be restricted on DWI/ADC sequences in solid parts. On post-contrast T1W images, MTs could be non-enhancing or show varying degree of contrast enhancement [4, 5, 7]. Malignant teratomas usually have heterogeneous marked enhancement on contrast enhanced T1WI, indicating vascular proliferation in the solid portion of the tumours. Therefore, marked enhancement of the solid portion or the thick wall of the tumour could be the key feature for distinguishing mature teratoma and malignant teratoma.

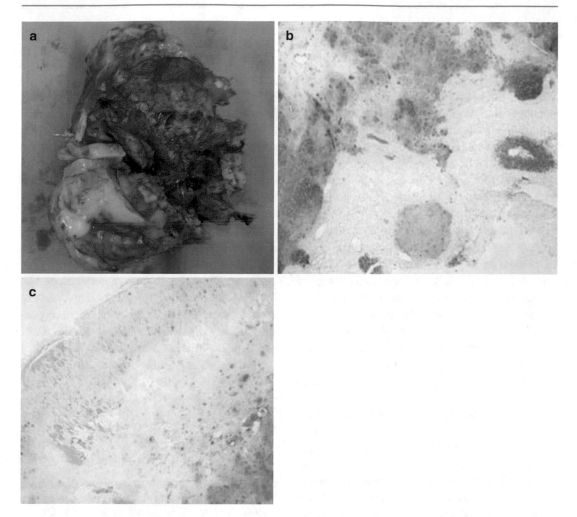

Fig. 4.3 Gross pathology of removed intracranial mature teratoma (**a**) (courtesy of D. Romić, specialist in neurosurgery). Microphotography of a pathohistological section of a removed teratoma stained with hemalaun eosin (courtesy of P. Sesar, specialist in pathology): cartilage and adipose tissue, magnification of ×40 (**b**); bone and cartilage, magnification of ×40 (**c**)

The majority of intracranial teratomas demonstrate at least some fat and some calcifications. Calcification can be found in half cases of mature teratomas, occasionally with mature bone or teeth [3, 5]. The high signal from fat on MRIs makes the identification of lipid easy.

MTs are usually without perilesional cerebral oedema on T2W images, due to the presence of tumours with capsules and undamaged blood–brain barrier.

It is important to exclude other intracranial neoplasms, commonly located in the pineal or suprasellar or parasellar region, before the diagnosis of teratoma is suggested. Differential diagnose includes other GCTs, craniopharyngioma, dermoid and epidermoid cyst due to its content and midline or para-midline location [5, 6, 7].

The patient's age and biochemical markers, such as serum AFP and β-HCG, can be useful in differentiating the lesions from other intracranial neoplasms. Serum AFP and β-HCG are useful biologic tumour markers characteristic of teratoma: elevated serum AFP levels are strongly indicative of malignant teratomas [4].

Pathohistological examination is the mainstay to establish a definitive diagnosis of an intracranial GCT.

Complete surgical resection is the gold standard for the treatment of intracranial MTs and generally shows no recurrence [8]. After surgical resection of MT, patients should be monitored by MRI for at least 10 years and more. It is because the occurrence of malignant teratoma or germinoma was found in adults and children several years and even after 10 or more years after total removal of a MT [8].

Our patient was a middle-aged female presenting with headache and large right frontal extra-axial parasagittal mass adhering to cerebral falx. A few very small, oval hypodensities at the lateral edge of the mass were mistaken for a CSF between the mass and the surrounding brain parenchyma on CT. Patient age, cerebral falx location, CT attenuation coefficients were misleading for radiologist who was thinking in the direction of a degenerated and calcified meningioma.

Small hypodensities at the lateral edge of the mass mistaken for a CSF on CT were hyperintense on T1WI due to fat. Tumour was mostly hyperdense on CT, but it was not due to meningeal origin or due to possible tumour hypercellularity: tumour was mostly hypointense on T1WI, T2WI and FLAIR and did not show decreased diffusion—it was due to its consisting components. From the standpoint of the MRI and CT findings, calcification and fatty components should have alerted radiologist to think of intracranial teratoma, and then it would be clear why most of the tumour showed hypointense signal on T1WI, T2WI, FLAIR FS and DWI sequences. It was obvious after the pathologist report: tumour consisted of mature cartilage tissue with some bone tissue that resulted in mostly hypointense signal. Tumour capsule showed only mild linear enhancement on post-contrast T1WI, and there was no vasogenic oedema in the surrounding frontal lobe parenchyma as previously mentioned.

Although tumour location in our patient was para-midline, cerebral falx is not a typical location for intracranial teratoma, but it is a possible one. Teratomas are generally thought to arise from misplaced primordial germ cells. Cerebral falx, cavernous sinus wall and septum pellucidum are histologically the same with dura mater. Therefore, abnormal migration of primordial germ cells into the dura mater might be responsible for the occurrence of interdural mature teratomas [1].

If you have a patient with an extra-axial mass in midline or para-midline region showing heterogeneous structure (solid or solid and cystic components) and heterogeneous densities on CT, look for calcifications and fatty components to confirm or exclude intracranial teratoma as possible diagnosis. Always take into consideration patient age and extra-axial mass location when considering other possible differential diagnosis.

References

1. Kong Z, et al. Central nervous system germ cell tumors: a review of the literature. J Child Neurol. 2018;33(9):610–20.
2. Louis DN, et al. The 2016 World Health Organization classification of tumors of the central nervous system: a summary. Acta Neuropathol. 2016;131:803–20.
3. Zhao J, et al. Cerebral falx mature teratoma with rare imaging in an adult. Int J Med Sci. 2012;9(4):269–73.
4. Filho PMM, et al. Intracranial mature teratoma: a case report. Arq Bras Neurocir. 2016;35:344–8.
5. Liu Z, et al. Imaging characteristics of primary intracranial teratoma. Acta Radiol. 2013;55(7):874–81.
6. Agrawal M, et al. Teratomas in central nervous system: a clinico-morphological study with review of literature. Neurol India. 2010;58(6):841–6.
7. Abdelmuhdi AS, et al. Intracranial teratoma: imaging, intraoperative and pathologic features. RadioGraphics. 2017;37:1506–11.
8. Lee YH, et al. Treatment and outcomes of primary intracranial teratoma. Childs Nerv Syst. 2009;25:1581–7.

Ruptured Dermoid Cyst and Ischaemic Stroke (After In-Vitro Fertilization Treatment)

At the beginning of January 2019, a 40-year-old female patient has woken up early in the morning feeling vertigo and tingling of the left hand. Symptoms did not diminish during the morning, and she came to our EHD where she was examined by a neurologist. In neurologist assessment ataxia, discreet left-sided hemiparesis and hypoesthesia were reported. Head CT was performed in the EHD and revealed ruptured dermoid cyst (Fig. 5.1). All laboratory findings, blood count, prothrombin time, C-reactive protein, urea, creatinine, electrolytes and liver function tests were normal on admission.

The patient was admitted to the hospital, and MRI of the brain was scheduled for the next day. Ruptured left temporal dermoid cyst was confirmed (Figs. 5.2 and 5.3), but MRI also revealed an acute ischaemia in the posterior limb of the right internal capsule and deep white matter above it (Fig. 5.4).

The patient was previously treated for hypothyroidism and was operated twice due to endometriosis. She was in gynaecologist treatment due to infertility and underwent in vitro fertilization (IVF) five times; latest IVF procedure was performed in November 2018 (about 2 months prior to this hospitalisation).

During her stay at neurology department, cardiologist and neurosurgeon were consulted. Electrocardiogram, 24-h Holter monitoring and echocardiography were normal. Neurosurgeon recommended surgical treatment of dermoid cyst

after conservative stroke treatment, out-hospital physical therapy was conducted, and the patient recovered.

Carotid and vertebral Doppler ultrasound was normal. She was also tested for thrombophilia: according to the result of testing, the patient was a heterozygous carrier for prothrombin G20210A mutation, or factor II mutation was found.

On discharge from the hospital, the patient had only discreet left-sided hemiparesis, and acetylsalicylic acid was recommended as therapy. Left-sided hemiparesis regressed entirely after physical therapy was conducted.

In April 2019, the patient underwent left pterional craniotomy, and content of the dermoid cyst was completely removed. Final pathologist report confirmed dermoid cyst: removed content of the cyst consisted of keratinaceous debris and detritus.

5.1 Ruptured Dermoid Cyst and Ischaemic Stroke (After In-Vitro Fertilization Treatment)

Intracranial dermoid cysts are rare non-neoplastic, congenital ectodermal inclusion cysts arising from the inclusion of ectodermal committed cells at the time of neural tube closure during the third to fifth week of embryonic life, accounting for up to 0.5% of all intracranial masses [1]. They are

M. Špero, H. Vavro, *Neuroradiology - Images vs Symptoms*,
https://doi.org/10.1007/978-3-030-69213-1_5

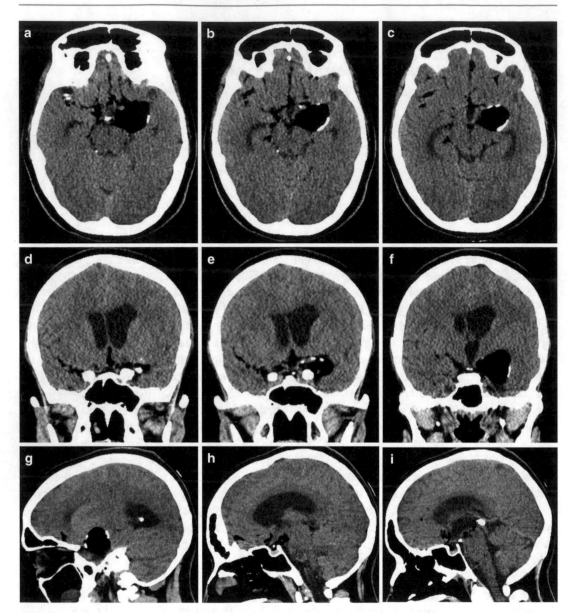

Fig. 5.1 Computed tomography of the brain, axial (**a–c**), coronal (**d–f**), sagittal (**g–i**), performed on admission revealed supratentorial left parasagittal temporal extra-axial mass: oval, well-circumscribed with a few linear calcification in the mass wall, homogenously hypodense–fat attenuating (about −66 Hu), consistent with dermoid cyst. There were multiple punctiform and small drops of fat diffusely in cerebral sulci on the basal aspect of the cerebral hemispheres (anterior and middle fossa), in suprasellar cistern, basal cisterns and in the frontal horn of the right lateral ventricle due to the ruptured dermoid cyst

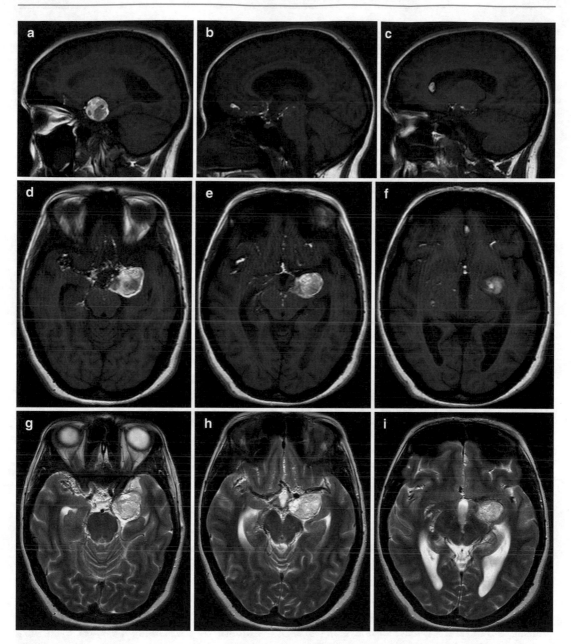

Fig. 5.2 Magnetic resonance imaging of the brain, sagittal T1WI (**a–c**), axial T1WI (**d–f**), T2WI (**g–i**), FLAIR FS (**j–l**), DWI (**m**), ADC (**n**), SWI (**o**), performed a day after the CT, confirmed diagnose of the ruptured dermoid cyst made on CT. The cyst was located at the left parasellar region extending to left temporal lobe, adjacent to mesial temporal part, which was slightly compressed by the cyst. Dermoid cyst was oval in shape, well-circumscribed, showed heterogeneous high signal on T1WI and T2WI, heterogeneous low signal on FLAIR FS, without restricted diffusion. There were evidence of rupture with fat signal droplets in the suprasellar cistern, basal cisterns, in cerebral sulci of the frontal lobes base, and frontal horn of the right lateral ventricle (**c**)

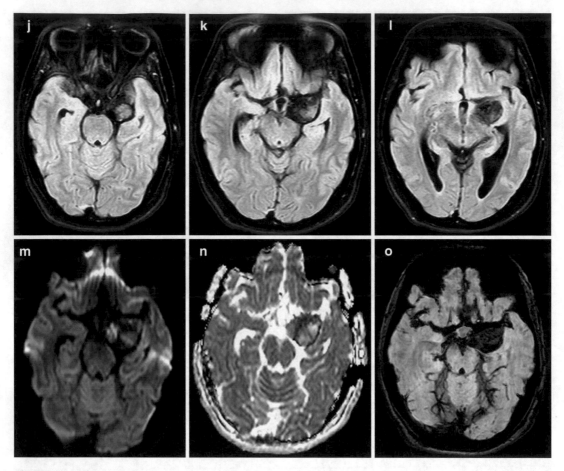

Fig. 5.2 (continued)

composed of mature squamous epithelium and contain varying amounts of ectoderm derivate including apocrine, sweat and sebaceous glands as well as hair follicles and possibly teeth [2].

They are most often found in midline sellar and suprasellar location, in parasellar and frontonasal region. Intracranial dermoids can also be found in the posterior cranial fossa. Supratentorial dermoid cysts (DCs) often present in the second or third decades of life, while posterior fossa dermoids typically present in the first decade of life as a consequence of mass effect exerted on the fourth ventricle with resulting hydrocephalus [2].

Dermoid cysts grow slowly in size due to the production of hair and oils from internal dermal elements, which results in increasing pressure. Therefore, DC presentation is variable. DCs may

remain asymptomatic and are found incidentally on CT or MRI performed for otherwise unrelated clinical complaints. Symptomatic DCs present with symptoms ascribed to mass effect on adjacent intracranial structures: headaches, seizures or rarely olfactory delusions [3, 4].

Rupture of intracranial dermoid cysts is a relatively uncommon phenomenon, usually spontaneous or following closed-head trauma. It results in dissemination of dermoid cyst content into the subarachnoid space and/or ventricles and meningeal irritation. Consequently, more serious complications such as aseptic chemical meningitis, vasospasm and cerebral infarction arise. Rarely, intra-ventricular fat leads to rapidly developing occlusive hydrocephalus. The mechanism of DC rupture is unknown: it is presumed that age-related hormonal changes may increase

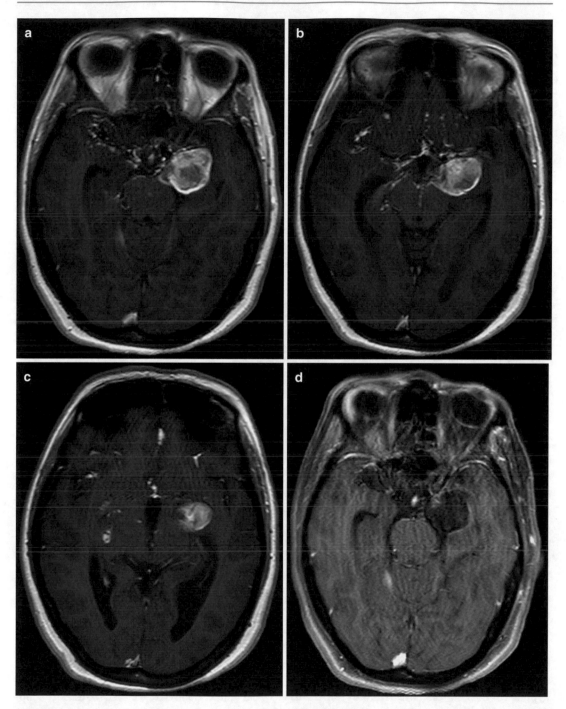

Fig. 5.3 Magnetic resonance imaging of the brain, post-contrast axial T1WI (**a–c**) T1FSWI (**d–f**). After intravenous administration of gadolinium contrast media T1FSWI revealed only thin rim of contrast enhancement in the dermoid cyst wall

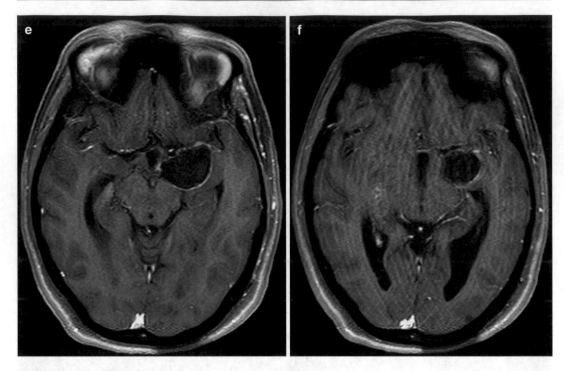

Fig. 5.3 (continued)

glandular secretions and lead to rapid expansion and rupture of these cysts [5–7].

The cyst content within the subarachnoid space can induce cerebral vasospasm or vasculitis which are considered as potential mechanisms of dermoid cyst rupture-related cerebral ischaemia. However, the hemodynamic mechanisms between cerebral ischaemia and DC rupture are not well known.

Symptom onset typically does not occur at the time of rupture, since the irritative effects of the spilled contents require time to develop and may also be delayed [4–7].

Imaging features of DCs on brain CT scans are pathognomonic. These cysts are usually rounded, well-circumscribed, extremely hypodense masses (negative Hu, 0 to −150 Hu) due to cyst lipid content. Peripheral capsular calcification is common, representing dystrophic changes or dental enamel, another ectodermal derivative. Generally, DCs do not show enhancement after contrast administration [1, 2, 4].

On MR images, dermoids are typically hyperintense on T1WI, heterogeneous on T2WI vary

from hypo- to hyperintense on FSE T2WI. Fat-suppression sequences can confirm the lipid presence within a lesion. DCs do not demonstrate restricted diffusion: DWI signal is hyperintense to brain parenchyma, but there is no signal loss on the ADC map. After gadolinium contrast administration, minimal enhancement of capsule is shown without central enhancement. DCs are never associated with vasogenic oedema. The "fat" density or signal seen in the images is not due to the presence of adipose tissue but depends on the internal composition of the lesion like cholesterol. Heterogeneous aspect depends on a keratinaceous debris, sebaceous and sweat secretion as well as appendages including hair and rarely nails or teeth [1, 3, 5, 6].

On both CT and MR images, fat-density droplets are seen throughout the subarachnoid space and in the ventricular system if rupture of the DC occurs. Leptomeningeal reaction and enhancement can be observed if DC rupture is complicated by chemical meningitis [5–7].

Rarely, dermoid cyst can show atypical or unusual appearance: on CT scans such DC is

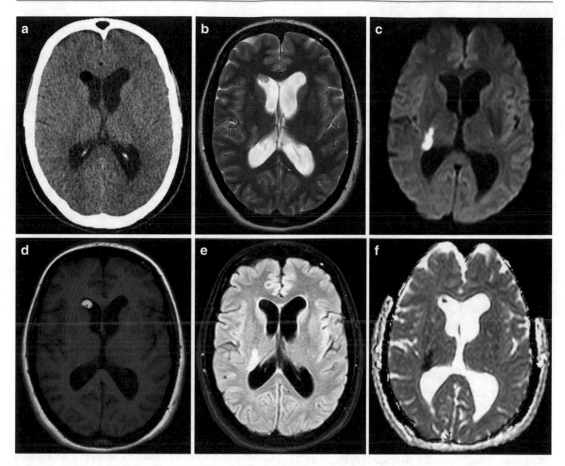

Fig. 5.4 Computed tomography of the brain on admission, axial (**a**): there was no evidence of acute ischaemia. Magnetic resonance imaging of the brain performed a day after the CT, axial T2WI (**b**), DWI (**c**), T1WI (**d**), FLAIR FS (**e**), ADC (**f**), revealed acute ischaemia in the posterior limb of the right internal capsule and deep white matter above it. Fat signal droplet in the frontal horn of the right lateral ventricle (**a**, **b**, **d**, **e**)

hyperdense, on MRI is hypointense on T1W and T2W images. It is thought to be due to combination of saponification of lipid/keratinized debris with secondary microcalcification in suspension, partially liquefied cholesterol, high protein content, and hemosiderin or iron–calcium complexes relating to previous episodes of haemorrhage within the cyst [4]. All of the reported CT hyper-attenuating dermoids have occurred in the posterior fossa, with no lesions ever having been identified supratentorially.

DC in our patient became symptomatic due to its rupture. Because of fertility problem she underwent IVF five times with the last IVF procedure performed about 2 months prior to the symptoms onset. Acute ischaemia became evident on MRI performed a day after the admission to hospital.

It was found that our patient was heterozygous carrier for prothrombin G20210A (factor II) mutation. Prothrombin is a precursor to thrombin, a key regulator of blood coagulation in the clotting cascade, and carriers of the prothrombin G20210A mutation have elevated blood plasma prothrombin levels. The prothrombin G20210A mutation has been associated with a two- to fourfold higher risk for venous thrombosis [8–10]. Jiang et al. have reported that the prothrombin G20210A mutation is associated with ischaemic stroke in young adults and may have an even higher association among the youngest group of young adults [8]. Specific to the population-based GEOS study, in adults with first ever ischaemic stroke before the age of 42 years, the prothrombin G20210A mutation may be a contributing factor [8]. According to results of the prospective study by Ricci et al., prothrombin G20210A mutation in asymptomatic women and in the absence of other risk factors is not associated with unexplained infertility and does not seem to affect IVF outcome [9].

In our opinion, hormonal changes due to IVF treatments may influence glandular secretions and lead to expansion and rupture of the DC. Acute ischaemia in this case could be the result of vasospasm induced by the spread of the DC content through subarachnoid space. Hypercoagulability due to the prothrombin G20210A mutation with increasing incidence of thromboembolic events should be taken into consideration as a possible contributing mechanism as well.

The most important differential diagnosis from other intracranial midline lesions includes epidermoid cyst, craniopharyngioma, teratoma and lipoma.

Appropriate treatment of DC is surgical resection: it may be subtotal resection since a DC is rarely followed by lesion recurrence [11].

References

1. Jackow J, et al. Ruptured intracranial dermoid cyst: a pictorial review. Pol J Radiol. 2018;83:465–70.
2. D'Amore A, et al. CT and MRI studies of giant dermoid cyst associated to fat dissemination at the cortical and cisternal cerebral spaces. Case Rep Radiol. 2013;2013(6):239258.
3. Kumran SP, et al. Unusual radiological presentation of intracranial dermoid cyst: a case series. Asian J Neurosurg. 2019;14:269–71.
4. Brown JY, et al. Unusal imaging appearance of an intracranial dermoid cyst. AJNR Am J Neuroradiol. 2001;22:1970–2.
5. Ballari S, Gurubharath I. Intracranial ruptured dermoid cyst presenting as dysarthria: a case report. IAIM. 2018;5(10):171–8.
6. Murrone D, et al. Ruptured intracranial dermoid cyst: a case report. Integr Mol Med. 2016;385:793–5.
7. Jin H, et al. Intracranial dermoid cyst rupture-related brain ischemia: case report and hemodynamic study. Medicine. 2017;96(4):e5631.
8. Jiang B, et al. The prothrombin G20210A mutation is associated with young-onset stroke: the genetics of early onset stroke study and meta-analysis. Stroke. 2014;45(4):961–7.
9. Ricci G, et al. Factor V Leiden and prothrombin gene G20210A mutation and in vitro fertilization: prospective cohort study. Hum Reprod. 2011;26(11):3068–77.
10. Fatini C, et al. Unexplained infertility: association with inherited thrombophilia. Thromb Res. 2012;129:185–8.
11. Orakcioglu B. Intracranial dermoid cysts: variations of radiological and clinical features. Acta Neurochir. 2008;150:1227–34.

A 49-year-old man had been suffering from lancinating facial pain in the area innervated by the first branch of the right-sided trigeminal nerve for almost 6 months before he decided to consult a physician. There was also occasional double vision. It had all started with occasional facial pain provoked by chewing or coughing.

Neurological status on initial exam: pain along the first branch (V1) and hypoesthesia in all three branch areas of the right-sided trigeminal nerve. Right abducens and right facial nerve hypofunction.

The patient was referred to an MRI of the brain with a diagnosis of a right-sided trigeminal neuralgia (Fig. 6.1).

The proposed diagnosis was a cystic degenerated schwannoma of the right-sided trigeminal nerve or an epidermoid cyst in the right Meckel's cave.

The patient underwent surgery via right-sided retro-mastoid approach which was uneventful, with achieved complete resection, the tumour was completely detached from the trigeminal nerve. The symptoms have resolved immediately after the surgery, only a mild facial numbness remained in the right V1 area.

The histopathology report stated vascular spaces of variable size and wall thickness containing red blood cells and thrombi, with surrounding reactive gliosis—findings consistent with a cavernous malformation (cavernoma).

6.1 Cavernous Malformation (CM) with Trigeminal Neuralgia

The most common cause of trigeminal neuralgia (TN) is microvascular compression, usually by superior cerebellar artery. Symptomatic neuralgia may be caused by herpes zoster, multiple sclerosis or neoplastic compression or involvement (e.g. schwannoma, meningioma, epidermoid). Only rarely TN occurs because of a cavernous malformation.

Cavernous malformations (CMs), also known as cavernomas or cavernous angiomas, consist of thin hyalinized vascular channels. They are low-flow vascular malformations which occur mostly in the brain, less often in the spinal cord and cranial nerves; they do not contain intervening brain or cord parenchyma [1].

The frequency of occurrence is proportional to parenchymal volume; hence, most of the CMs are found in the supratentorial brain. There are case reports on CMs affecting optic nerve and chiasm, oculomotor nerve, facial nerve and vestibular nerve. There are less than 20 reports of trigeminal nerve involvement.

Extra-axial CMs are very rare, thought to develop from capillary plexuses related to the dura mater and are mostly found at the floor of the middle cranial fossa, especially in the cavernous sinus [2]. They are somewhat different from

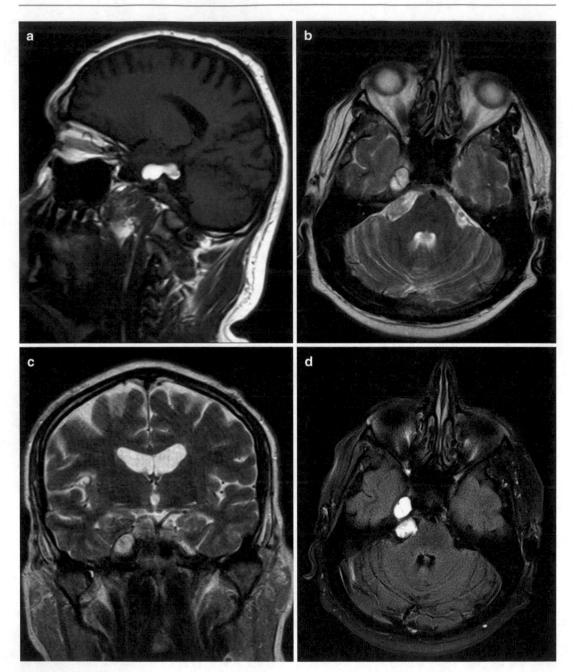

Fig. 6.1 MRI exam of the brain—sagittal T1WI (**a**), axial (**b**) and coronal (**c**) T2WI, axial T2-FLAIR image (**d**), axial SWI images (**e, f**), axial CISS image (**g**) with coronal (**h**) and sagittal (**i**) reformats. An hourglass-shaped mass lesion in the right-sided prepontine cistern and Meckel's cave. A large segment of the right trigeminal nerve seems to be dislocated laterally and cranially, it is not clearly visible. Note the peripheral hemosiderin in the lesion seen in (**e**) and several small hemosiderin-laden lesions in the bilateral brain parenchyma in (**f**) which may represent cavernomas (see Chap. 17)

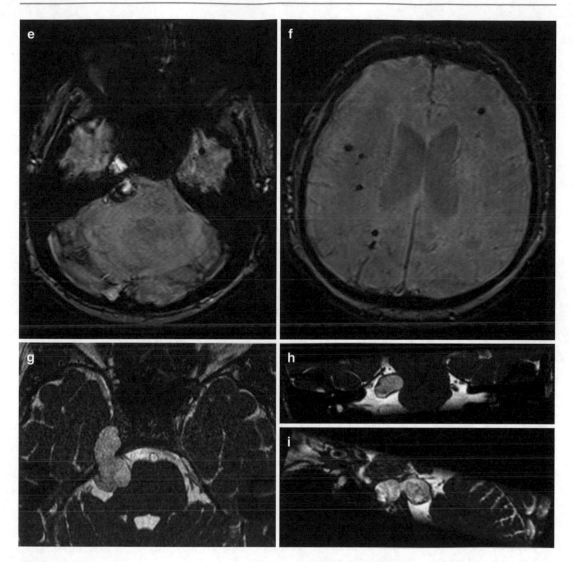

Fig. 6.1 (continued)

the intra-axial lesions on CT and MRI and may be misdiagnosed as meningiomas [3].

CMs are found in 0.4–0.8% of the population. They make 10–25% of all CNS vascular malformations, being surpassed in frequency only by developmental venous anomalies (DVAs, venous angiomas) which are often found in association with CMs.

On imaging, CMs affecting trigeminal nerve may lack some of the obvious imaging features of CMs described in Chap. 1 of this book, such as "popcorn" appearance or a clear hemosiderin rim, especially in types G and C (see below). There may be cystic degeneration such as in this case, probably caused by repetitive small contained haemorrhages. The differential diagnoses included in the initial MRI report of this case were cystic schwannoma (would be hypointense in T1WI, with peripheral contrast enhancement, diffusion not compromised) and epidermoid cyst (usually isointense to CSF in T1WI and T2WI).

Establishing CM location is essential for treatment planning. The treatment of choice is surgery aiming at complete resection since incomplete excision may increase the risk of haemorrhage; surgical approach depends on CM location [2].

CM causing trigeminal neuralgia may have its origin in:

- The Gasserian ganglion (Type G)—develops from the dural or cranial nerve vascular plexus.
- The cisternal portion up to the intra-axial portion of the trigeminal nerve root (Type C)—

develops from the vascular plexus of the cranial nerve.

- In the intra-axial trigeminal nerve root in the pons (Type P)—develops from the parenchymal vascular plexus.
- In the spinal tract of the trigeminal nerve root (Type S)—develops from the parenchymal vascular plexus [2].

There is also a possibility of stereotaxic radiosurgical therapy with one case report [4] of pain relief by approximately 75%. On the other hand, there are reports of radiation-related complications and haemorrhage which occur in up to 40% of cases treated by stereotaxic radiosurgery.

References

1. Batra S, et al. Cavernous malformations: natural history, diagnosis and treatment. Nat Rev Neurol. 2009;5(12): 659–70. https://doi.org/10.1038/nrneurol.2009.177.
2. Adachi K, et al. A review of cavernous malformations with trigeminal neuralgia. Clin Neurol Neurosurg. 2014;125:151–4. https://doi.org/10.1016/j.clineuro.2014.07.025.
3. Kanaan I, et al. Extra-axial cavernous hemangioma: two case reports. Skull Base. 2001;11(4):287–95. https://doi.org/10.1055/s-2001-18635.
4. Pease M, et al. Gamma knife radiosurgery for trigeminal neuralgia caused by a cavernous malformation: case report and literature review. Stereotact Funct Neurosurg. 2018;96(6):412–5. https://doi.org/10.1159/000495476.

Aortic Pseudoaneurysm Eroding Thoracic Spine

In 2018, a 70-year-old male patient presented with worsening of the back pain followed by haemoptysis. Back pain was more pronounced while sitting and walking, ceased in the supine position. Neurological symptoms were not present.

A year before, thoracic endovascular aortic repair (TEVAR) was performed due to descending thoracic aorta pseudoaneurysm which was diagnosed at the chest and abdominal CT performed (Fig. 7.1) due to the elevated sedimentation rate, 51 mm/h (normal range 3–23 mm/h): white cells blood count was within the normal range. The patient was treated with risedronate and vitamin D for osteoporosis with fracture of the sixth and tenth thoracic vertebrae discovered on chest and abdominal CT. He had a history of chronic bronchitis and arterial hypertension.

CT of the aorta was performed in the EHD on the admission (Fig. 7.2) and MRI of the thoracic and lumbar spine was recommended in the report. CT revealed well-corticated erosion of the ninth thoracic vertebral body, no evidence of endoleak or aortic stent–graft migration (Fig. 7.2), as well as no evidence of pseudoaneurysm enlargement in comparison to previous CT.

The first follow-up CT of the aorta was performed 3 months after TEVAR and did not reveal evidence of the ninth vertebral body erosion as well as no difference in high and shape of the sixth and tenth vertebral body after the chronic osteoporotic fracture (Fig. 7.3a, d). The next follow-up CT was performed 8 months after the procedure and 10 months before this hospitalization in 2018: it revealed small erosion of the anterior aspect of the ninth thoracic vertebral body (Fig. 7.3b, c, e, f) which demonstrated significant increase in size in comparison to the CT performed at the emergency admission (Fig. 7.2).

MRI of the thoracic and lumbar spine confirmed bone erosion due to the descending thoracic aorta pseudoaneurysm (Figs. 7.4 and 7.5).

Percutaneous bone biopsy was performed and pathohistological logical finding was in concordance with chronic osteomyelitis, while bacterial and fungal cultures after bone biopsy were negative. Diagnostic work-up during hospitalization also included bronchoscopy and neck and chest CT due to haemoptysis. Bronchoscopy did not reveal active bleeding or evidence of endobronchial obstruction. Neck and chest CT did not demonstrated neoplastic process, but there were minor reactive changes due to pseudoaneurysmal compression in the adjacent left lung parenchyma thought to be the cause of the haemoptysis.

Orthopaedic surgeon did not indicate surgical stabilization of the thoracic spine, but a thoracic lumbar sacral orthosis (TLSO) as a conservative method to stabilise the spine.

M. Špero, H. Vavro, *Neuroradiology - Images vs Symptoms*,
https://doi.org/10.1007/978-3-030-69213-1_7

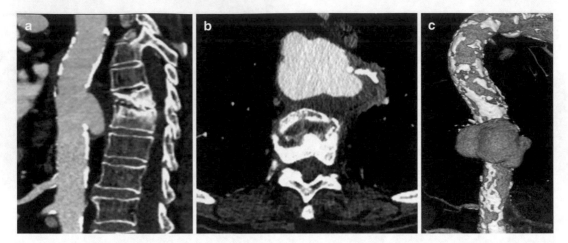

Fig. 7.1 Chest and abdominal computed tomography (2017), post-contrast, sagittal (**a**) and axial (**b**) scans, volume rendering (**c**), performed due to an elevated sedimentation rate, revealed descending thoracic aorta pseudoaneurysm extending in front of the ninth, tenth and eleventh thoracic vertebrae with the loss of fat plan separating the pseudoaneurysm from the anterior aspect of the adjacent thoracic vertebrae. Chronic osteoporotic anterior wedge fracture of the tenth thoracic vertebral body and degenerative changes at Th9–Th10 and Th10–Th11 level, more pronounced at Th10–Th11 level. Afterward, TEVAR was performed to treat pseudoaneurysm

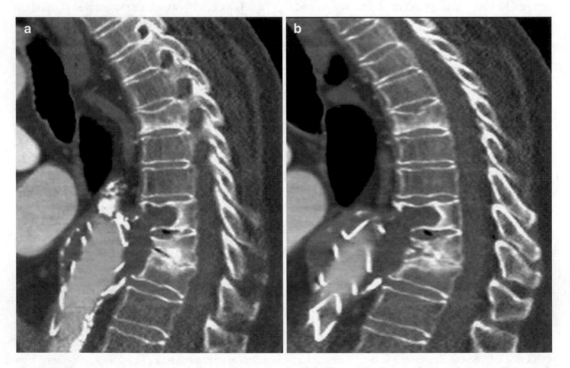

Fig. 7.2 Computed tomography of the aorta, post-contrast, sagittal (**a**, **b**) and axial (**c**, **d**) scans, revealed well-corticated erosion of the ninth thoracic vertebral body described as osteolysis. There was no evidence of endoleak or aortic stent–graft migration, as well as no evidence of pseudoaneurysm enlargement in comparison to previous CT performed 10 months earlier

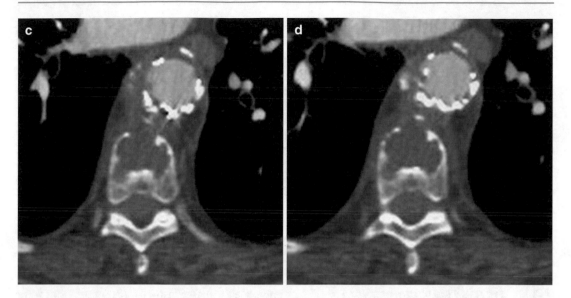

Fig. 7.2   (continued)

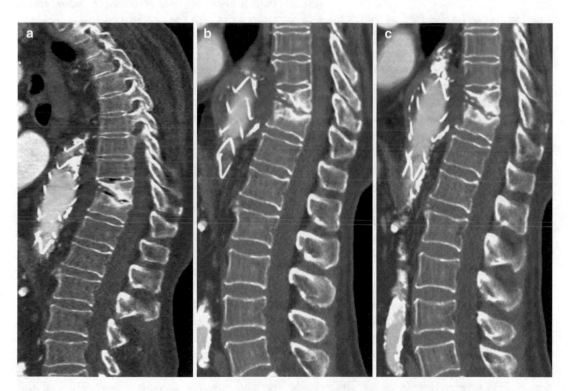

Fig. 7.3 Post-contrast computed tomography of the aorta, performed 3 months after TEVAR, sagittal (**a**) and axial (**d**) scans, did not reveal evidence of the ninth vertebral body erosion. CT of the aorta performed 8 months after the procedure, sagittal (**b**, **c**) and axial (**e**, **f**) scans, revealed small erosion of the anterior aspect of the ninth thoracic vertebral body

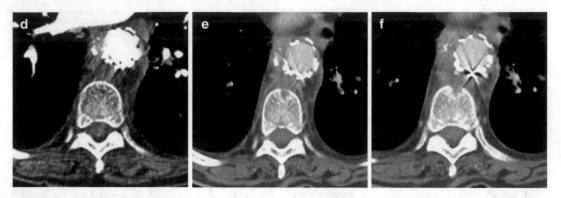

Fig. 7.3   (continued)

7.1   Aortic Pseudoaneurysm Eroding Thoracic Spine

Aneurysms can be classified as true or false. In a true aneurysm, all three layers of the vessel wall are present (intima, media and adventitia). In a false aneurysm, or pseudoaneurysm, an opening in one of the vessel wall layers allows the leakage of blood through its wall, which is subsequently contained by scar tissue or the adventitia itself: such a type of an aneurysm is usually caused by trauma or prior surgery [1].

Vertebral body erosion secondary to a thoracic or abdominal aortic aneurysm is an uncommon but important cause of back pain.

Such vertebral erosions are most often located in the anterior aspect of the vertebral body and usually do not exceed 50% of it, occurring in 7% to more than 25% of the cases [2]. Generally, they are due to vascular prosthesis infections, chronic, contained aneurysm rupture or expansion. There are two suggested pathophysiological mechanism of thoracic or abdominal aneurysm complicated with vertebral erosion. The first is a repetitive mechanical pressure by arterial pulsation causing relative bone ischemia, which leads to lysis and bone destruction/remodelling marked with cortical sclerosis: osteoporosis increases the risk of erosion. The second mechanism is a direct extension of vertebral osteomyelitis or discitis to involve the aorta and cause mycotic aortic aneurysm formation. Infection and inflammation are

not uncommon. Most of these aneurysms are mycotic in nature, often tuberculous. The most common organisms identified in aortic and vertebral lesions are *Mycobacterium tuberculosis*, *Salmonella* species, Gram-positive cocci and Gram-negative bacilli excluding *Salmonella* [3–5].

Clinical presentation of vertebral erosions due to aortic aneurysm usually includes fatigue, weight loss, fever, localized chronic back pain and neurological deficits (paraparesis or paraplegia) [6].

CT angiography of the aorta is the reference examination. It allows studying the whole thoraco-abdominal aorta and its branches and assessing the relationship with the different adjacent structures including retroperitoneal structures, psoas muscles and thoracic and lumbar spine. This method makes it possible to evaluate the signs of aneurysmal rupture, intra- or retroperitoneal haematoma and predictive signs of rupture, such as rupture of the continuity of parietal calcifications or the draped aorta sign which refers to the loss of fat plan that separates aorta from the anterior aspect of the spine and psoas muscle. Erosion of the anterior aspect of vertebral body is the amplest manifestation of this sign. Magnetic resonance imaging may be indicated in stable patients for comparative monitoring of lesions, assessment of possible involvement of neural structures, evaluation of spondylitis or spondylodiscitis because it detects oedema within the trabecular bone very early, before the

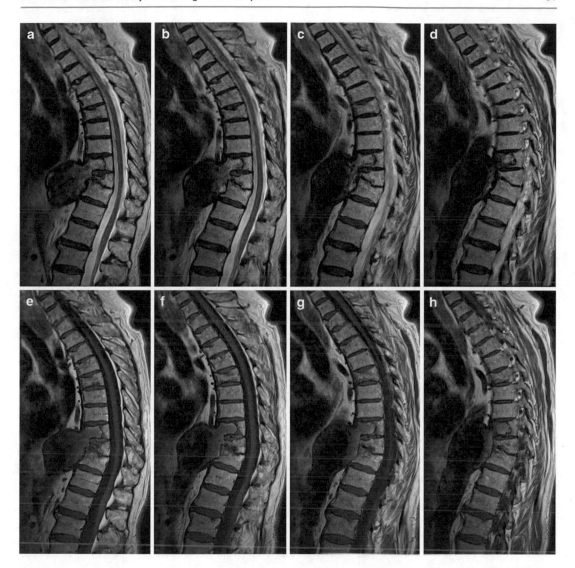

Fig. 7.4 Magnetic resonance imaging of the thoracic and lumbar spine, non-contrast sagittal T2WI (**a–d**), T1WI (**e–h**), STIR (**i–l**), and post-contrast sagittal T1WI (**m–p**), demonstrated descending thoracic aorta pseudoaneurysm that measured 6.5 cm by 5.1 cm in the greatest dimensions on the axial view, treated by TEVAR and well-corticated erosion of the ninth thoracic vertebral body which was normal in height. There was no evidence of adjacent bone oedema or contrast enhancement of the bone. Intervertebral discs at the Th9–Th10 and Th10–Th11 levels demonstrated desiccation in setting of degenerative changes with narrowing of Th9–Th10 and Th10–Th11 space and irregular vertebral body endplates. Chronic osteoporotic anterior wedge fracture of the tenth thoracic vertebral body and more pronounced degenerative changes at the Th10–Th11 level were present

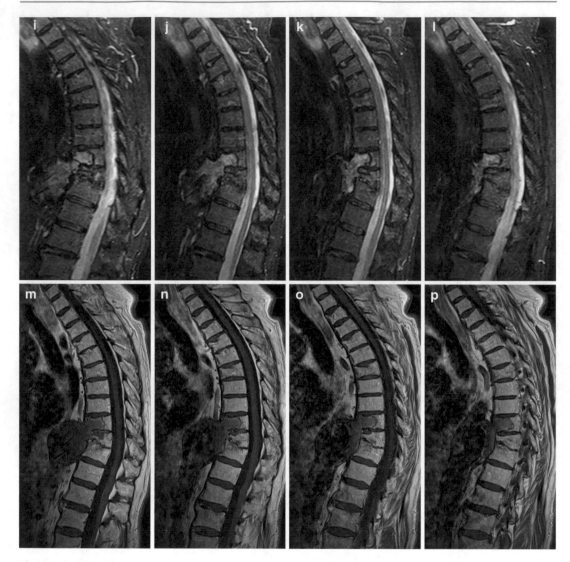

Fig. 7.4 (continued)

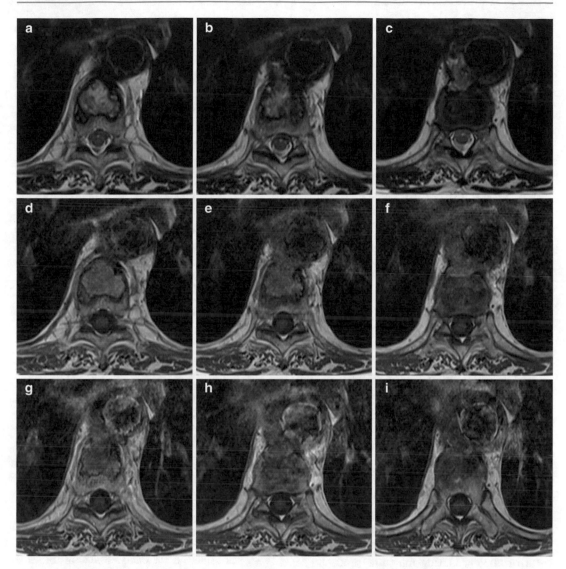

Fig. 7.5 Magnetic resonance of the thoracic spine, non-contrast axial T2WI (**a–c**) and T1WI (**d–f**), and post-contrast axial T1WI (**g–i**), demonstrated the extent of bone erosion involving more than two thirds of the anterior aspect of the ninth thoracic vertebral body and sclerotic margins of the erosion. The ninth thoracic vertebral body was normal in size and shape, and the rest of the vertebral body had normal signal intensities

onset of destruction. Preservation of the disk spaces on CT decreases the risk of infection and helps in making differential diagnosis [2, 6–8]. Image-guided percutaneous spine biopsy and bacterial and mycotic cultures are important in infection evaluation.

The pseudotumoral aspect of bone erosion can direct radiologist towards a tumour (metastasis, multiple myeloma) or infectious (tuberculosis) origin. Vertebral collapse and lytic lesions are usually related to fractures, tumours, osteoporosis, spondylitis or spondylodiscitis. In contrast with other mycotic aortic aneurysms, most cases of tuberculous aortic aneurysms are diagnosed on the basis of histopathology without culture confirmation.

Radiologists should keep in mind possible aortic aneurysm or pseudoaneurysm as a cause of vertebral erosions involving the anterior aspect of the vertebral body in differential diagnosis [8].

Endovascular aortic aneurysm repair (EVAR) was first described in 1991 [9]. Since that time, it has been established over open surgical repair as the preferred method for treating abdominal aortic aneurysms in patients with suitable anatomy, given its slower mortality rate and comparable long-term survival. Aortic graft infection as a complication of EVAR is a relatively rare problem, with an incidence of 0.5–1% [10].

In case of a severe vertebral destruction, orthopaedic stabilization of the spine is the treatment of choice. During the same procedure, if needed, vascular reconstruction could be performed as well. If neurological symptoms are not present, conservative treatment for stability fixation could be applied [8, 10].

Regarding this patient, it was unclear from the beginning what was the aetiology of its descending thoracic aorta pseudoaneurysm that was treated by TEVAR. On CT and MRI, tenth thoracic vertebral body demonstrated anterior wedge shape due to a chronic osteoporotic fracture. Endplates of the Th10 and Th11 vertebrae were slightly irregular in shape and sclerotic, intervertebral disc space at the Th10–Th11 level was markedly narrow (Figs. 7.2 and 7.4). Such changes could be a result of potential, previously unrecognized discitis which could have extended towards aortic wall causing aortitis. Unrecognized aortitis could have resulted in pseudoaneurysm extending in front of ninth, tenth and eleventh thoracic vertebrae. Descending thoracic aorta pseudoaneurysm was treated with EVAR, while bone erosion of the anterior aspect of the ninth vertebral body appeared about 8 months after the procedure (Fig. 7.3b, c, e, f). In the absence of trauma in anamnesis, such scenario could have explained pseudoaneurysm aetiology and vertebral body erosion (Figs. 7.4 and 7.5) as a complication after TEVAR in the patient.

References

1. Lombardi AF, et al. Extensive erosion of vertebral bodies due to a chronic contained ruptured abdominal aortic aneurysm. Radiol Case. 2016;10(1):27–34.
2. Toufga Z, et al. Vertebral erosion secondary to aortic aneurysm. Case Rep Radiol. 2020;2020:1–3.
3. Wansink J, van den Kleij FGH. Vertebral-body erosion in thoracic aortic aneurysm. N Engl J Med. 2016;374:9.
4. Rajab TK, et al. Aortic aneurysm eroding into the spine. Aorta. 2018;6:68–9.
5. Takahashi Y, et al. Descending thoracic aortic aneurysm complicated with severe vertebral erosion. Eur J Cardiothorac Surg. 2007;31:941–3.
6. Forutan H. Paraparesis due to pressure erosion of the thoracic spine by an aortic aneurysm: remission of symptoms following resection of the aneurysm and vertebral reconstruction. Acta Neurochir. 2004;146:303–8.
7. Zanini LA, et al. Vertebral body erosion secondary to aortoiliac aneurysm. Einstein. 2019;17(4):eAI4550.
8. Mandegaran R, et al. Spondylodiscitis following endovascular abdominal aortic aneurysm repair: imaging perspectives from a single centre's experience. Skelet Radiol. 2018;47:1357–69.
9. Parodi JC, Palmaz JC, Barone HD. Transfemoral intraluminal graft implantation for abdominal aortic aneurysms. Ann Vasc Surg. 1991;5:491–9.
10. Nesmachnyy A, et al. Surgical treatment for chronic-contained rupture of thoracic aortic aneurysm complicated with vertebral erosion: case report. Ann Clin Case Rep. 2017;2:1425.

Two years prior to being admitted to our hospital, this 48-year-old woman had had a surgery for a spinal epidural arachnoid cyst of the lower dorsal region in another facility because of long-standing pain in lower back and left leg. Unfortunately, the pain persisted after the surgery. The previous imaging had been unavailable, so we had do to the imaging work-up without comparative analysis. The available medical documentation stated a prior T12 laminectomy and fenestration of an arachnoid cyst at T12–L1 level.

EMG and nerve conducting study showed signs of severe neuronal lesion in the muscles of the left calf and foot.

An MRI exam of the lumbar spine and thoracic–lumbar junction was requested (Fig. 8.1).

Neurosurgical opinion was that conventional MR imaging did not suffice, so MR myelography was requested (Fig. 8.2).

Additionally, a CT myelography requested by the neurosurgeons demonstrated communication of the cyst with the spinal CSF space (Fig. 8.3).

The patient underwent a second surgery—the cyst was evacuated, the pain has resolved, but not completely. On follow-up MRI, there was a small residual extradural cyst measuring 10×20 mm.

8.1 Spinal Extradural Arachnoid Cyst

Spinal extradural arachnoid cysts (SEACs) develops from arachnoid mater herniating through small dural defects—they contain CSF as there is a communication with the intradural CSF space through a small pedicle. The dural defect is most often located in the region of the dural sleeve of the spinal nerve root—the assumed mechanism is stretching across relatively mobile dural sleeve and fixed nerve root. The rootlet then may act as a ball-valve, allowing further filling of the SEAC but preventing CSF from leaking out of the cyst, effectively causing enlargement [1]. They are most probably congenital, but can be acquired from trauma, infection or inflammation. The congenital origin theory is supported by their frequent association with diastematomyelia, neural tube defects, syringomyelia, spina bifida, multiple sclerosis and Marfan syndrome. There are also reports of familial cases with loss of *FOXC2* gene function, supporting genetic aetiology. Apart from the ball-valve mechanism, the proposed expansion mechanisms cystic are active secretion of liquid through the cyst walls (but

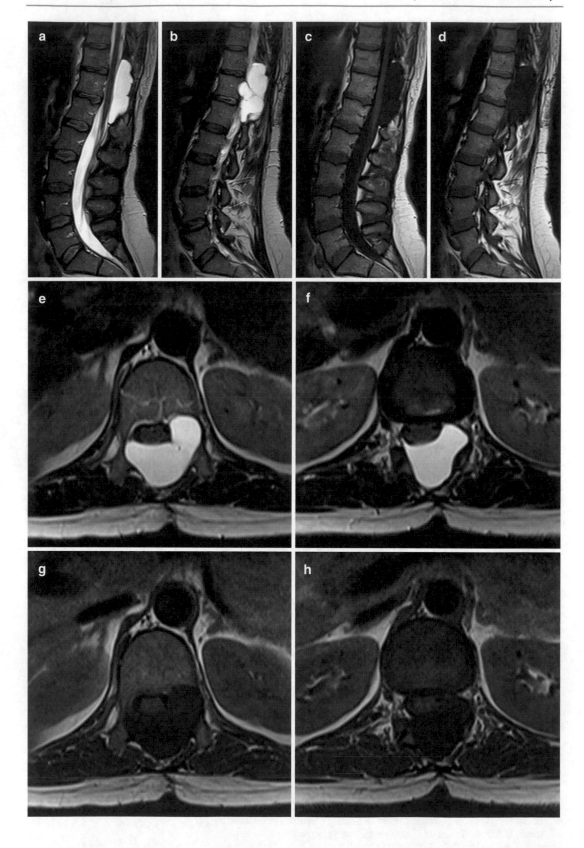

there are no histopathologic findings to support that), passive osmosis of water and hydrostatic pressure of cerebrospinal fluid [2].

SEACs are a rare cause of thecal sac and spinal cord compression, accounting for only 1% of spinal tumours. Men are affected twice more commonly than women [3]. The most common location is middle to lower thoracic spine (65%), followed by lumbar and lumbosacral (13%), thoracolumbar (12%), sacral (7%) and cervical regions (3%) [3]. Thoracic cysts are more common in adolescents, while thoracolumbar and lumbar cysts occur in adults in the fourth decade of life. They arise dorsally and can protrude into neural foramens, as in this case.

The symptoms produced by SEACs depend on the severity and location of compression. Cervical cysts may cause spastic tetraparesis and sensory impairment; Horner syndrome occurs with low cervical cysts; thoracic cysts present with progressive spastic paraparesis but usually no pain, while the leading presenting symptom of lumbar and lumbosacral cysts is low-back pain, radiculopathy and bladder and bowel dysfunction [4]. Approximately 30% of patients experience remission and fluctuation of symptoms which in some cases can be exacerbated by Valsalva manoeuvre.

Classification of spinal meningeal cysts brought by Nabors et al. [5] puts SEACs into group 1a (spinal extradural meningeal cysts without nerve root fibres).

Histologically, the SEAC wall is composed of layers of collagenous fibres and a membrane with flat lining cells—no secretory cells are present.

On MR imaging, SEAC follows the CSF signal intensity; in T2WI, it is possibly brighter because there are no pulsation signal loss artefacts. It does not enhance with intravenous gadolinium contrast. Most often it is sited in the posterior, and/or posterolateral aspect of the spinal canal (most cases are unilateral), anteriorly bordered by dura, unilaterally invaginating into neural foramina; the scalloping of the posterior vertebral elements and enlargement of the foramina suggests a long-standing process with an increased hydrostatic pressure. Conventional MRI may not demonstrate the communication between the intradural space and SEAC, even using sub-millimetre high-resolution sequences. CSF flow-sensitive sequences may demonstrate a pulsating flow-void at the site of communication [1].

CT myelography is a tool to prove the neurosurgeons that MRI report describing a SEAC is actually accurate, as it can demonstrate accumulation of the iodine contrast medium in the SEAC and thus confirm its communication with intradural subarachnoid space, such as in case described in this chapter. However, do not expect it to enable you to pinpoint the exact site of communication. Also, post-contrast imaging should be delayed to allow enough time for the contrast to accumulate in the cyst. Some authors scan immediately and then 3 hours or 8 hours later, and the next morning [4]. In the light of reducing the CT radiation dose, a single scan several (e.g. 4) hours after intrathecal application of the appropriate iodine contrast media should be enough to demonstrate contrast in the cyst.

Treatment in asymptomatic cysts consists of regular imaging follow-ups. In symptomatic patients, surgery is the mainstay of treatment. Lately many authors advocate tailored laminectomy and fenestration of the cyst with utmost importance of repairing the dural defect to prevent recurrence, as opposed to multiple laminectomies for complete cyst resection [1]. In order to minimize surgically inflicted damage, advanced imaging with the ultimate aim of demonstrating the communication between the intradural subarachnoid space and SEAC is essential.

Fig. 8.1 MRI exam of the thoracic–lumbar junction. Sagittal T2WI (**a**, **b**), sagittal T1WI (**c**, **d**), axial T2WI (**e**, **f**) and axial T1WI (**g**, **h**). There is evidence of previous laminectomy at T11 and T12. An extradural cystic mass is seen in the posterior and left lateral aspect of the spinal canal at T11 to L1, compressing and dislocating the dural sac and distal thoracic spinal cord and remodelling the left posterior aspect of the body and left pedicle of the T12 vertebra, extending into the left neural foramen. The findings are consistent with a spinal extradural arachnoid cyst

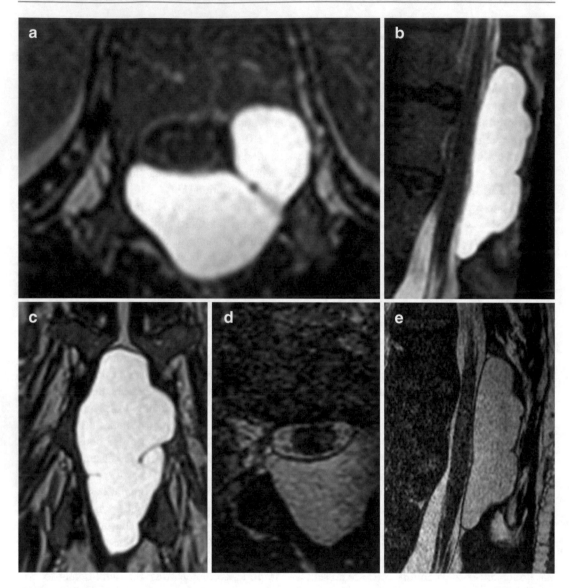

Fig. 8.2 MR myelography, T2W axial 0.9 mm image (**a**) with sagittal (**b**) and coronal (**c**) reformats. Compare with axial (**d**) and sagittal (**e**) 0.6 mm CISS images which show dura in more detail. No obvious communication between the cyst and spinal subarachnoid space

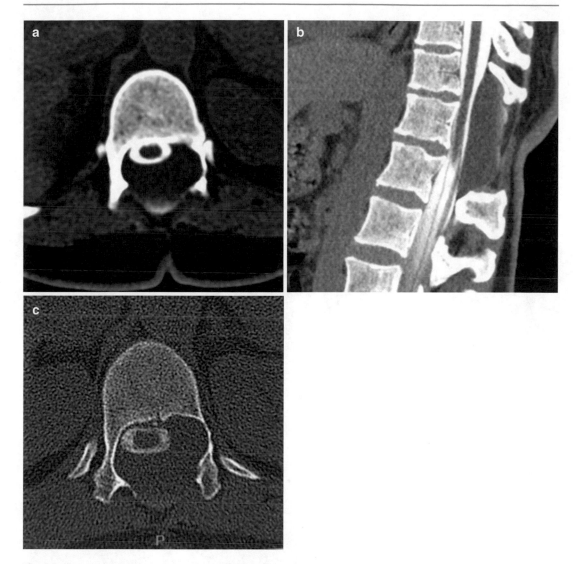

Fig. 8.3 CT myelography, supine position of the patient. A layer of intrathecally applied iodine contrast medium is seen dependent in the posterior aspect of the cyst (**a**, **b**), confirming communication of the cyst and spinal CSF space, but without an obvious site of leak. Bony reconstruction algorithm shows the extent of T12 vertebral remodelling (**c**). Note the previous T12 lamiectomy

References

1. Choi SW, et al. Spinal extradural arachnoid cyst. J Korean Neurosurg Soc. 2013;54(4):355–8. https://doi.org/10.3340/jkns.2013.54.4.355.
2. Quillo-Olvera J, et al. Quiste aracnoideo extradural espinal: reporte de un caso y revisión de la literatura [spinal extradural arachnoid cyst: a case report and review of literature]. Cir Cir. 2017;85(6):544–8. https://doi.org/10.1016/j.circir.2016.09.003.
3. Cloward RB. Congenital spinal extradural cysts: case report with review of literature. Ann Surg. 1968;168(5):851–64. https://doi.org/10.1097/00000658-196811000-00011.
4. Liu JK, et al. Spinal extradural arachnoid cysts: clinical, radiological, and surgical features. Neurosurg Focus. 2007;22(2):E6. https://doi.org/10.3171/foc.2007.22.2.6.
5. Nabors MW, Pait TG, Byrd EB, et al. Updated assessment and current classification of spinal meningeal cysts. J Neurosurg. 1988;68(3):366–77. https://doi.org/10.3171/jns.1988.68.3.0366.

Spinal Intramedullary Ependymal Cysts

9

A 62-year-old female patient was examined in the EHD due to positional vertigo with nausea and neck pain.

Eleven months ago, she underwent right mastectomy and axillary clearance due to invasive breast carcinoma (no special type, NST, grade 2, luminal B). Five months ago, radiation therapy was conducted, while adjuvant chemotherapy was ongoing at the time.

Brain CT performed in the EHD was unremarkable, and neurologist recommended MRI of the cervical spine. In neurologist assessment, there was no motor lateralization, but the patient described discreet intermittent right arm tingling.

After analysing MRI of the cervical spine, I reported spinal intramedullary ependymal cyst (Fig. 9.1). There was no evidence of metastatic lesion in the cervical spine due to beast malignant tumour she was treated for. Neurosurgeon was consulted. He recommended follow-up MRI of the cervical spine which was performed in 3 months and did not reveal changes in shape, size or signal intensity of the spinal intramedullary cyst. Surgical treatment has not been recommended for the time being.

9.1 Intramedullary Ependymal Spinal Cyst

Intradural ependymal spinal cysts are rare, like other developmental intradural cysts, while spinal intramedullary ependymal cysts are particularly rare, representing 0.4% of all primary spinal tumours [1]. Hyman et al. first reported a patient with intradural ependymal cyst in 1938 [2], while Mosso and Verity classified ependymal cysts into intradural extramedullary, intramedullary and mixed variety in 1975 [3].

Ependymal cysts are a thin-walled cysts pathologically characterized by a lining of columnar or cuboidal epithelium, with or without cilia, that lacks a basement membrane and rests on glial tissue. The cyst cavity is usually filled with clear serous fluid secreted by ependymal cells [4, 5].

Spinal ependymal cysts are of developmental origin. The most widely accepted hypothesis regarding the genesis of these cysts states that the floor plate of the neural tube is invaginated on the ventral side and becomes isolated to form an ependymal cyst later. The location of the isolated ependymal cells determines whether the cyst is

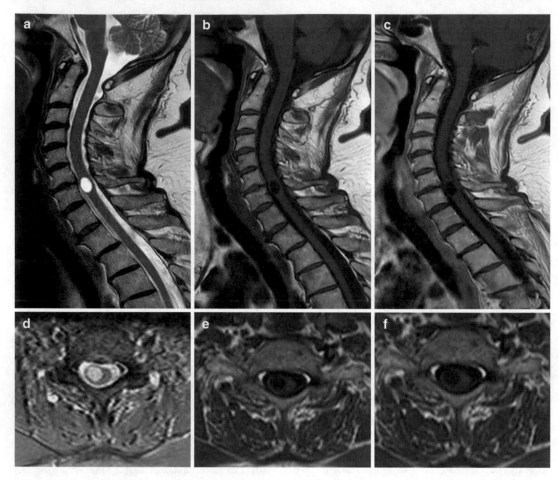

Fig. 9.1 Magnetic resonance imaging of the cervical spine, non-contrast sagittal (**a**) and axial (**d**) T2WI, sagittal (**b**) and axial (**e**) T1WI, and post-contrast sagittal (**c**) and axial (**f**) T1WI-revealed slightly expansile lesion in the right part of the spinal cord at the C6–C7 levels. Intramedullary lesion was oval, well-circumscribed, slightly enlarging right part of the spinal cord. Lesion itself was hyperintense on T2WI (**a**, **d**), hypointense on T1WI (**b**, **e**), followed CSF signal intensities. It did not show contrast enhancement on post-contrast T1WI (**c**, **f**). There was no perilesional oedema, as well as no enlargement of the central canal of the spinal cord (hydromyelia) or syrinx

present intramedullary or extramedullary; also this may cause the cyst to be present anywhere along the craniospinal axis. The central canal too has a lining of ependymal cells, but they do not form a cyst, because the secretion of these lining cells of the central canal are either absorbed or flow along with CSF, while the isolated ependymal cells have their secretions collecting and thus forming a cyst [4, 5].

Spinal intramedullary ependymal cysts are described in children and adults, twice are commoner in females occurring in the age group of 38–71 years. They may arise at all levels of the spinal cord from cervical to the conus, while conus medullaris is the most frequent site [4]. According to the literature, variable presenting symptoms have been reported depending on the site and size of the cyst. Clinical presentation of spinal intramedullary ependymal cysts include intermittent paraparesis, quadriparesis, radicular pain, extremity numbness and paresthesias. The symptoms onset is usually gradual, the course is progressive.

MRI is the imaging method of choice for evaluating and differentiating spinal cord cysts.

Spinal intramedullary ependymal cysts appear as well-circumscribed lesions with thin, smooth wall causing focal expansion of the spinal cord extending over involved segments. Cysts are located off-centre from the central canal and involve anterior, dorsal or lateral part of the spinal cord, usually located on the anterior cord, without perilesional oedema. They are hypointense on T1WI, hyperintense on T2W and STIR images following CSF signal intensities. After intravenous administration of gadolinium contrast medium, there is no contrast enhancement [4, 5]. The MRI diagnosis of ependymal cyst relies on the exclusion of other conditions that may lead to cystic changes in the spinal cord such as the Chiari malformation, other anomalies of the craniovertebral junction, posttraumatic cyst, neoplastic lesions, and the ventriculus terminalis in case of a conal location [4]. Clinical history, non-central location and confined nature of the cyst are important radiological findings useful for differentiating such cysts from congenital or traumatic cystic spinal cord lesions. Lack of contrast enhancement on MRI allows its differentiation from neoplastic lesions. Ventriculus terminalis is a congenital cystic dilatation in the midline conus usually seen in the paediatric age group: the off-central location of the cyst, no association with spinal dysraphism and non-paediatric onset of the symptoms predispose the diagnosis of ependymal cyst.

Pathological diagnosis after the MRI will confirm diagnose. Ultrastructural and immunocytochemical staining features have been recently described and allow histological differentiation of a spinal intramedullary ependymal cyst from other cysts.

In symptomatic cases, treatment is surgical. The aim of surgical treatment is cord decompression and prevention of the cyst from refilling, which is best accomplished by completely resecting the cyst and closing the communication between the cyst and the subarachnoid space. Because the cyst wall usually cannot be separated from the cord parenchyma, the only possible treatment is creating communication between the cyst and the subarachnoid space by means of fenestration or marsupialization [5, 6].

The nature of this lesion is benign and usually shows partial or complete recovery of function with a low recurrence rate. Although there are no clear guidelines for the interval of follow-up in the literature, close MRI follow-up is recommended in order to exclude recurrence (despite rare) or an unexpected evolution [5].

Spinal intramedullary ependymal cyst was accidental finding in a case of our patient. She was in neurologist treatment due to vertigo and neck pain, and I presume the MRI was recommended to exclude possible secondary malignant involvement or possible disk herniation—there was no sign of both, but the described cystic spinal cord lesion was found. Because the patient had only intermitted right arm tingling and was under the oncologic treatment neurosurgeon did not recommend surgical treatment at the time. Surgical treatment will probably be taken into consideration after the oncology treatment is completed and if the symptoms progress. Although this is, for now, pathologically unconfirmed case, all radiomorphological characteristics fit into the diagnosis: lesion looks the same as the pathologically confirmed, spinal intramedullary ependymal cysts published in the literature by now.

References

1. Figueiredo F, et al. Spinal intramedullary ependymal cyst – current concepts for diagnosis and surgical management Brit. J Neurosurg. 2014;28(3):406–7.
2. Hyman I, et al. Ependymal cyst of the cervicodorsal region of the spinal cord. Neurol Psychiatry. 1938;40:1005–10127.
3. Mosso JA, Verity MA. Ependymal cyst of the spinal cord. Case report. J Neurosurg. 1975;43(6):757–60.
4. Saito K, et al. Spinal intramedullary ependymal cyst: a case report and review of the literature. Acta Neurochir. 2005;147:443–6.
5. Park CH, et al. Spinal intramedullary ependymal cysts: a case report and review of the literature. J Korean Neurosurg Soc. 2012;52:67–70.
6. Iwahashi H, et al. Spinal intramedullary ependymal cyst: a case report. Surg Neurol. 1999;52:357–61.

Pilocytic Astrocytoma at the L1–L2 Level

In 2018, a 50-year-old male patient came for MRI of the lumbar spine as an outpatient. MRI was recommended by neurologist due to bilateral, mainly left-sided radiculopathy with radicular pain and weakness in the left leg lasting for several months (Fig. 10.1).

I reported intradural extramedullary spinal tumour: due to L1–L2 levels location, signal intensities and inhomogeneous appearance on all sequences, I presumed it could be degenerated Schwannoma.

Patient underwent L1 laminectomy, Th12 and L2 laminotomy and tumour biopsy. Final pathologist report was pilocytic astrocytoma grade I according to 2016 WHO classification: the diagnosis was confirmed on light microscopy and immunohistochemistry. Surgical procedure was without complication. After postoperative physical therapy, the patient had intermittent pain in the right leg, without any other symptom. Residual tumour was described on the first postoperative follow-up MRI of the lumbar spine (Fig. 10.2).

10.1 Pilocytic Astrocytoma at the L1–L2 Level

Primary spinal astrocytoma is a subtype of glioma, the second most common spinal cord tumour found in the intradural intramedullary compartment. Spinal astrocytomas account for 6–8% of all spinal cord tumours [1]. Subtypes of astrocytomas include pilocytic astrocytoma (PA), diffuse astrocytoma, anaplastic astrocytoma and glioblastoma multiforme (grade IV astrocytoma or malignant glioblastoma).

According to the 2016 WHO classification of CNS tumours, PA represents grade I tumours histologically [2]. These are benign tumours of low to moderate cellularity with loosely textured areas, consisting of multipolar cells, microcapsules, and eosinophilic granular bodies, as well as densely fibrillated areas rich in Rosenthal fibres, composed of cells with long bipolar processes and elongated cytologically bland nuclei [3].

PA is the most common CNS glioma in the paediatric and adolescent population, uncommon in adults, usually younger adults (about 30 years old), without sexual predilection [4]. These are slow growing neoplasms with predominantly indolent behaviour, and the symptoms can take months to years to present. PAs of the spine are almost exclusively intramedullary in location with a low recurrence rate and an excellent prognosis following complete surgical resection [5, 6].

Purely intradural extramedullary astrocytomas are extremely rare, in the region of medullary conus and cauda equina accounting for only 4% of all spinal astrocytomas [1], with very few cases reported in the literature. It has been postulated that extramedullary gliomas likely arise

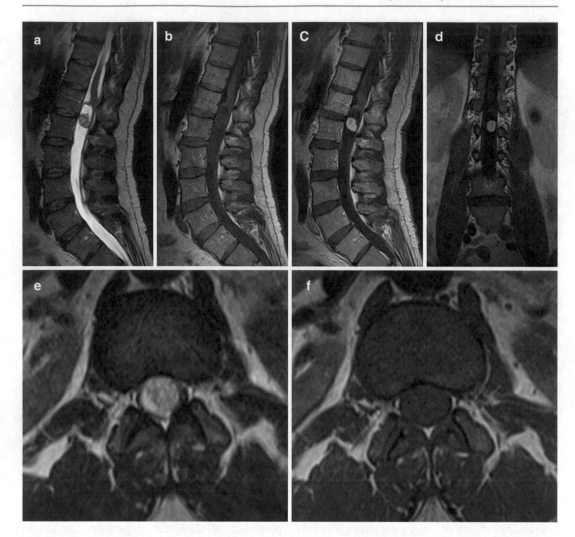

Fig. 10.1 Magnetic resonance imaging of the lumbar spine, T2WI sagittal (**a**) and axial (**e, h**), non-contrast T1WI sagittal (**b**) and axial (**f, i**), post-contrast T1WI sagittal (**c**), coronal (**d**) and axial (**g, j**), revealed intradural extramedullary mass at the L1–L2 levels, distal to conus medullaris. Within the dural sac mass was located in the midline, and bilateral para-midline, more left side. It appeared like mass was attached to one nerve root within cauda equina roots, hanging from it, while conus medullaris was slightly pushed upwards. Mass was round in shape, demonstrated slightly inhomogeneous signal on non-contrast sequences, mainly iso- to hyperintense on T2WI and iso- to hypointense on T1WI. On post-contrast T1WI, it demonstrated inhomogeneous contrast enhancement. Post-contrast T1WI in sagittal plane of the cervical and thoracic spine did not reveal any other spinal lesion

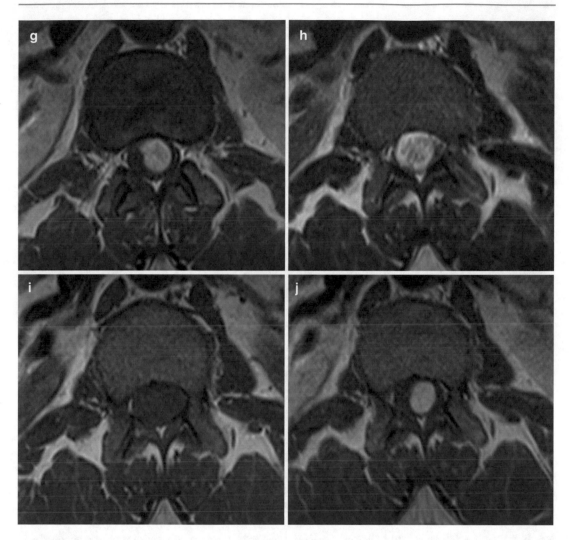

Fig. 10.1 (continued)

from heterotopic glial nests in pia and arachnoid membranes: Wolback first drew attention to the presence of glial heterotopias in 1907 [6, 7].

The first published presentation of intradural extramedullary astrocytoma was by Cushing and Eisenhardt in 1938: they reported spinal intradural extramedullary glioma which looked like a meningioma but on histopathology was found to be astrocytomas [8]. Later on, in 1951 Cooper et al. reported 15 cases of extramedullary gliomas; nine of these were intradural of which five were astrocytoma, two were in thoracolumbar region [9], while Wilkinson and Mark in 1968

reported a case of thoracic extramedullary astrocytoma [10].

Clinical symptoms are non-specific, including local or less frequently irradiating pain. Motor weakness and bowel and bladder dysfunction sometimes only present in the later stage of the disease, thereby delaying the diagnosis [11].

MRI of the lumbar spine, with and without gadolinium, is the imaging method of choice. On MRI, astrocytomas are usually hypo- to isointense on T1WI and hyperintense on T2WI. They present as focal enlargements of the spinal cord originating eccentrically from cord parenchyma

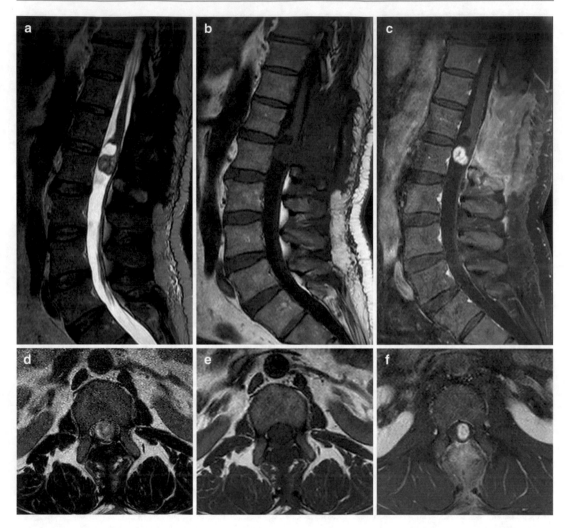

Fig. 10.2 The first follow-up MRI of the lumbar spine, T2WI sagittal (**a**) and axial (**d**), non-contrast T1WI sagittal (**b**) and axial (**e**), post-contrast T1WI FS sagittal (**c**) and axial (**f**), revealed residual tumour a bit smaller in size, which did not show changes in signal intensities or contrast enhancement pattern

within the posterior cord. Despite the fact they are low grade, nearly all spinal astrocytomas show some level of enhancement on post-contrast T1W images [3, 4]. Cysts are a common finding of spinal astrocytomas. These cysts are usually intratumoural, and most of them have peripheral contrast enhancement (lining of a syrinx does not show contrast uptake). Tumour margins are irregular and not always clearly defined: after gadolinium administration, tumour is usually better delineated from oedema, cysts and syrinxes [4].

We have presented a case of an intradural extramedullary pilocytic astrocytoma independent of a primary intraparenchymal tumour in an adult patient with no history of pilocytic astrocytoma.

The radiographic differential diagnosis for intradural extramedullary tumours in this anatomic location is commonly meningioma or nerve sheath tumours.

After analysing MRI of the lumbar spine, I reported intradural extramedullary spinal tumour. Due to tumour anatomic location at cauda region, tumour appearance as it was attached to a nerve root within it, signal intensities and inhomogeneous appearance on non-contrast and post-contrast sequences, although it was not pronouncedly hyperintense on T2WI, I presumed it could be a slightly degenerated schwannoma. The histopathological report surprised us with the diagnosis being pilocytic astrocytoma, which was clear on light microscopy and confirmed on immunohistochemistry.

As I have already mentioned, intradural extramedullary astrocytomas are extremely rare tumours, especially in the conus-cauda region. Therefore, taking location into consideration as well, they are easily mistaken for a nerve sheath tumours in cauda equina region. Since those tumours are rare, there is no specific MRI appearance of intradural extramedullary astrocytomas published in the literature. All reported intradural extramedullary PA had different radiological appearance. For example, Singh P et al. reported well demarcated intradural mass at L2, lying to the left of conus that was isointense to the conus in T1WI and isointense to CSF in T2WI [12]. Winstein et al. reported intradural, extramedullary mass at L1–L2 levels and presumed it was schwannoma: non-contrast MRI showed intrinsic T1 hypointensity and heterogeneous T2 hyperintensity, and post-contrast imaging showed homogenous post-contrast enhancement. Final pathohistological finding revealed low-grade glial neoplasm, with histologic features of ependymoma and pilocytic astrocytoma, closely intermixed, collision tumour [13]. Kumar A et al. reported giant cystic intradural extramedullary PA of cauda equina extending from L4 to S4 [1].

The management of pilocytic astrocytomas of spinal cord involves surgery with or without adjuvant radiation therapy. As these lesions are benign, patients can be followed up after surgery, and radiation therapy can be applied in a case of recurrence or regrowth [1].

This case as well as other reported cases of intradural extramedullary PA in conus-cauda region emphasizes the need to consider pilocytic astrocytoma in the differential diagnosis of cauda equina tumours.

References

1. Kumar A, et al. Giant cystic intradural extramedullary pilocytic astrocytoma of Cauda equina. J Neurosci Rural Pract. 2013;4(4):453–6.
2. Louis DN, et al. The 2016 World Health Organization classification of tumors of the central nervous system: a summary. Acta Neuropathol. 2016;131(6):803–20.
3. She DJ, et al. MR imaging features of spinal pilocytic astrocytoma. BMC Med Imaging. 2019;19:5.
4. Basheer A, et al. Multifocal intradural extramedullary pilocytic astrocytomas of the spinal cord: a case report and review of the literature. Neurosurgery. 2017;80:178–84.
5. Benes V, et al. Prognostic factors in intramedullary astrocytomas: a literature review. Eur Spine J. 2009;18(10):1397–422.
6. Helseth A, Mørk SJ. Primary intraspinal neoplasms in Norway, 1955 to 1986. A population-based survey of 467 patients. J Neurosurg. 1989;71(6):842–5.
7. Cooper IS, Kernohan JW. Heterotopic glial nests in the subarachnoid space; histopathologic characteristics, mode of origin and relation to meningeal gliomas. J Neuropathol Exp Neurol. 1951;10(1):16–29.
8. Cushing H, Eisenhardt L. Meningiomas, their classification, regional behaviour, life history and surgical results. Springfield: Chalrles C Thomas; 1938. p. 785.
9. Cooper IS, et al. Tumours of spinal cord primary extramedullary gliomas. Surg Gynecol Obstet. 1951;92:183–90.
10. Wilkinson IIA, Mark VH. Thoracic extramedullary astrocytoma: case report. J Neurosurg. 1968;28:504–8.
11. Koeller KK, et al. Neoplasms of the spinal cord and filum terminale: radiologic-pathologic correlation. Radiographics. 2000;20:1721–49.
12. Singh P, et al. Extramedullary astrocytoma of conus region: a short report. Neurol India. 2001;49(1):97–9.
13. Weinstein GM, et al. Spinal intradural, extramedullary ependymomawith astrocytoma component: a case report and review of the literature. Case Rep Pathol. 2016;2016:3534791.

At the moment of consulting a neurologist in our facility, this 54-year-old man had been suffering from intermittent headaches for 2 years, with no other health problems. He did not take any medications. No focal neurological symptoms were present. EEG demonstrated diffusely irregular findings, with slower waves in both frontal-temporal regions, more on the right. A head CT exam was called for, showing a heavily calcified infratentorial lesion (Fig. 11.1).

After the CT report had been done, the patient was referred to head MRI for further analysis (Fig. 11.2).

No surgical action was recommended as this was thought to be an incidental finding of CAPNON.

Follow-up MRIs 7.5 months and 2 years after the initial MRI did not demonstrate any change in lesion appearance (Fig. 11.3).

11.1 Calcifying Pseudoneoplasm of the Neuraxis (CAPNON)

As one can guess from its name, calcifying pseudoneoplasm of the neuraxis is a non-neoplastic, calcified lesion which can occur anywhere in the central nervous system. Also called fibro-osseous lesion of the neuraxis and CRUDoma, it is a very rare lesion with fewer than 100 cases reported since the first in 1978; it occurs in both adults and children without a specific sex predilection [1]. The main histological feature is chondromyxoid fibrillary matrix, which may be nodular, interlacing linear or amorphous in appearance. Potential histological features are spindled or epithelioid cells palisading around the matrix, variable fibrous stroma, ossification, psammoma bodies and foreign-body giant cells, while calcification is found in majority of cases [1, 2]. Calcification is more frequent in the intracranial and skull base cases; spinal lesions tend to be smaller at presentation. The chondromyxoid matrix is not invariably present. Fibroblasts are thought to be involved in its production; abnormal adjacent cartilage is a frequent finding [1].

The aetiology of CAPNON is not completely clear—at first, it was thought to be idiopathic and sporadic, but with more pathological insight, a suspicion of concurrent or underlying pathology evolved. Considered aetiology was reactive proliferative and metaplastic transformation [3]. It has been reported in association with inflammatory, degenerative and vascular pathologies, prior trauma or infection and neoplasms, both benign and malignant [1, 4]. Concomitantly found lesions include meningoangiomatosis, DNET, meningioma, low-grade glioma and ependymoma [1]. In general, it is agreed that CAPNON represents a benign reactive lesion that may develop as a response to inciting factors such as trauma, infection, inflammation or degeneration [1].

CAPNON is usually solitary, although multiple lesions have been described [3]. The presenting symptoms depend on location, size

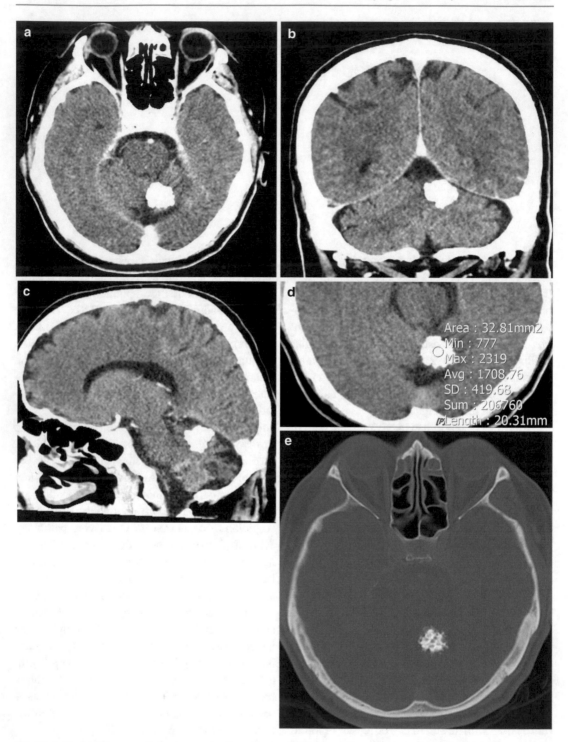

Fig. 11.1 Brain CT exam. Contrast-enhanced (**a–c**) and non-contrast (**d**) images, with a bony reconstruction algorithm image (**e**), showing a heavily calcified lesion (1700 HU) in the left cerebellar vermis, measuring 22 × 19 × 18 mm, without an appreciable mass effect or abnormal contrast accumulation

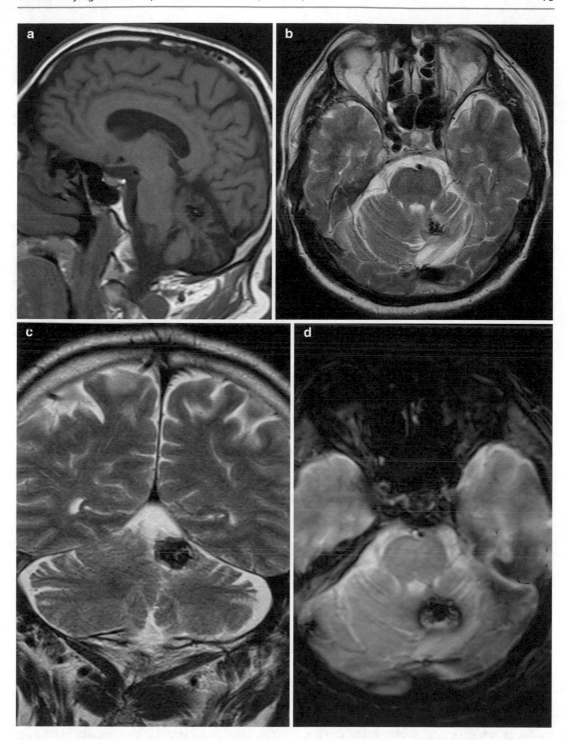

Fig. 11.2 Brain MRI. Sagittal T1WI (**a**), axial (**b**) and coronal (**c**) T2WI, axial SWI (**d**), axial T2-FLAIR (**e**) and axial contrast-enhanced T1WI (**f**), showing a slightly lobulated mass in the left cerebellar vermis, mildly inhomo- geneous but mostly hypointense in T1WI and T2WI, with a narrow rim of gliosis and contrast enhancement. No evidence of significant mass effect

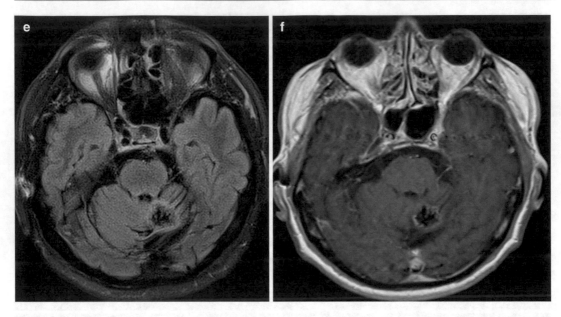

Fig. 11.2 (continued)

and mass effect exerted on neural structures and include pain, seizures and focal sensory and motor impairment. Intracranial lesions have been found in the dura, brain parenchyma, corpus callosum, ventricles, pineal gland, cisternal spaces and at the foramen magnum. Orbits, sella, clivus, temporal bone and cranial nerves may also be affected. Spinal lesions were reported at the cervical, thoracic, lumbar and sacral segments and may involve facet joints, intervertebral discs, dura, neural foramina and spinal cord [1].

On imaging, CAPNON usually appears as diffusely or coarsely calcified leptomeningeal or parenchymal mass on CT. Heavily calcified, well-defined parenchymal or leptomeningeal lesion without or with minimal perifocal oedema, uniformly low-intensity in T1WI and T2WI, without solid enhancement is a classic appearance of a CAPNON. T2WI may demonstrate variable degrees of mixed signal, but usually with a hypointense rim [4, 5], making it difficult to differentiate from a calcified neoplasm or a cavernoma. There may be subtle internal or rim contrast enhancement [1, 2]. On SWI, there is

marked hypointensity with mild blooming. Dural attachments are frequent. If present, bone remodelling features smooth bone margins, without erosions and destruction [1].

Differential diagnoses include cavernous malformation (cavernoma), meningioma (especially at the skull base), oligodendroglioma, ganglioglioma and astrocytoma with calcifications. Intraventricular CAPNON should be distinguished from choroid plexus tumours, ependymal tumours and meningioma [2]. Calcified infectious lesions (neurocysticercosis, tuberculosis) should also be considered [4]. In the spine, bone tumours, disc degeneration and degenerative synovial cysts may show overlapping features [1].

Surgical resection is the treatment of choice in symptomatic CAPNON, with no reports of recurrence if gross total resection is achieved. Although rare, CAPNON should be recognized as a possible diagnosis when heavily calcified lesions hypointense in both T1WI and T2WI are found, without significant enhancement and perifocal oedema, to avoid unnecessary invasive procedures.

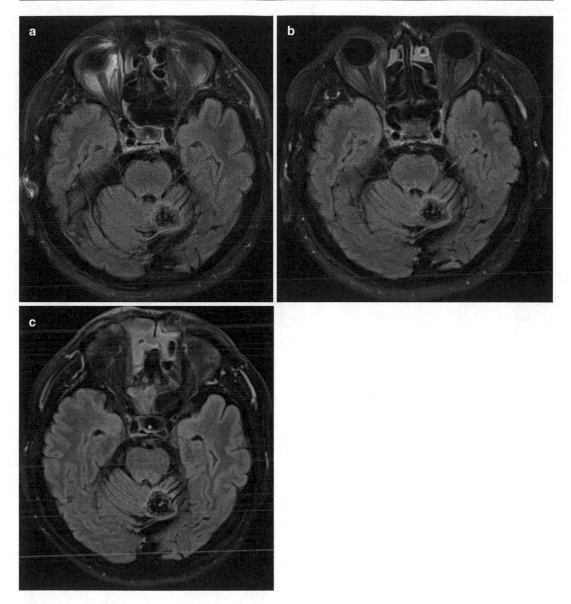

Fig. 11.3 T2-FLAIR MR images of the brain. Comparison of initial (**a**), first follow-up (7.5 months later, **b**) and second follow-up (2 years after initial exam, **c**) images. No evidence of change in CAPNON appearance

References

1. Ho M-L, et al. New insights into calcifying pseudoneoplasm of the neuraxis (CAPNON): a 20-year radiological-pathological study of 37 cases. Histopathology. 2020;76(7):1055–69. https://doi.org/10.1111/his.14066.
2. Aiken AH, et al. Calcifying pseudoneoplasms of the neuraxis: CT, MR imaging, and histologic features. AJNR Am J Neuroradiol. 2009;30(6):1256–60. https://doi.org/10.3174/ajnr.A1505.
3. Brasiliense LB, et al. Multiple calcifying pseudoneoplasms of the neuraxis. Cureus. 2017;9(2):e1044. https://doi.org/10.7759/cureus.1044.
4. Pithon RFA, et al. Calcifying pseudoneoplasm of the neuraxis. Radiol Bras. 2019;52(5):342–3. https://doi.org/10.1590/0100-3984.2017.0171.
5. Tanoue Y, et al. Surgically treated intracranial supratentorial calcifying pseudoneoplasms of the neuraxis (CAPNON) with drug-resistant left temporal lobe epilepsy: a case report and review of the literature. Epilepsy Beh Case Rep. 2019;11:107–14. https://doi.org/10.1016/j.ebcr.2019.02.002.

Part II

Epileptic Seizure

Antiphospholipid Syndrome in a Patient with Systemic Lupus Erythematosus Elements

In 2019, a 52-year-old female patient was hospitalized due to diagnostic work-up of suspected antiphospholipid syndrome and suspected lupus nephritis.

In 1997, she was diagnosed with epilepsy due to a grand mal epileptic seizures: according to a written MRI report changes related to a possible CNS vasculitis were described, while CSF findings were normal. According to medical documentation, brain MRI was performed in 2016 and 2017: did not reveal changes in number, size and signal intensities of previously reported lesions consistent with possible CNS vasculitis. The patient was under neurologist supervision during past 20 years, and this was her first contact with immunologist although its consultation was previously recommended by neurologist. In 2018, anticardiolipin IgG and IgM were positive while anti-beta-2-glycoprotein 1 antibody was negative.

She had a history of two unexplained spontaneous abortion, in the first and second trimesters, and two successful pregnancies. In the first pregnancy, she suffered from gestational diabetes, and during the second one, she was taking low dose of acetylsalicylic acid. Her recommended medication therapy included antiepileptic medications and acetylsalicylic acid, and from 2017 antihypertensive medication due to arterial hypertension.

The patient was presented with frontal and occipital headaches sometimes followed with diplopia lasting for several years. She denied pain or swelling of the joints, mucosal ulceration or dryness, cold fingers or toes, colour changes in skin in response to cold or stress, previous arterial or venous thrombosis.

Laboratory findings revealed normal CRP and sedimentation rate, mild thrombocytopenia, normal APTV, normal levels of urea and creatinine, proteinuria (1.79–2.14 g in 24-h urine) with normal urine sediment findings, decreased complement component 3 and 4, positive antinuclear antibodies, positive dsDNA antibodies, positive anticardiolipin IgG and IgM, positive lupus anticoagulant and positive beta-2-glycoprotein 1 antibody.

Renal biopsy confirmed thrombotic microangiopathy. MRI of the brain and cerebral MRA were performed as well. Cerebral MRA did not reveal changes of large cerebral arteries consistent with large vessel vasculitis. Brain MRI confirmed gliotic changes in the setting of chronic vascular lesions possibly consistent with antiphospholipid syndrome: in comparison with MRI, from 2017, there were no changes in number, size or signal intensities of reported lesions (Fig.12.1). There were no evidence of cerebral microbleeds on SWI or contrast enhancement on post-contrast T1 MPRAGE.

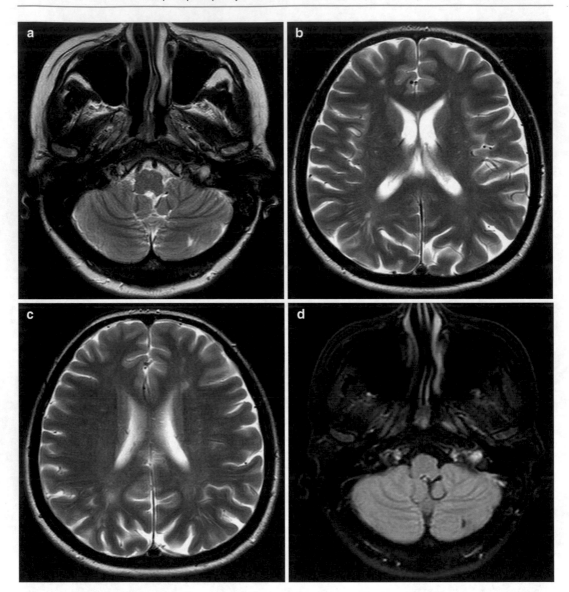

Fig. 12.1 MRI of the brain, non-contrast axial T2WI (**a–c, g–i**) and FLAIR FS (**d–f, j–l**) revealed supratentorial bilateral multifocal, oval and linear white matter hyperintensities in frontal and parietal lobes and one old lacunar lesion in the posterior part of left cerebellar hemisphere (**a, d**). Mild parietal postcentral atrophy

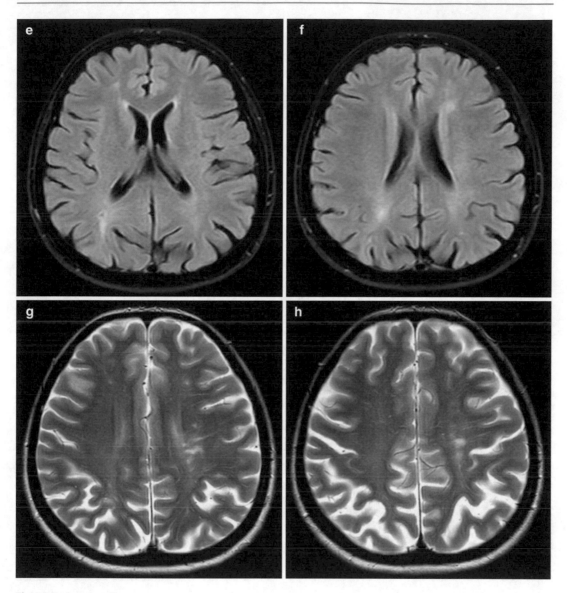

Fig. 12.1 (continued)

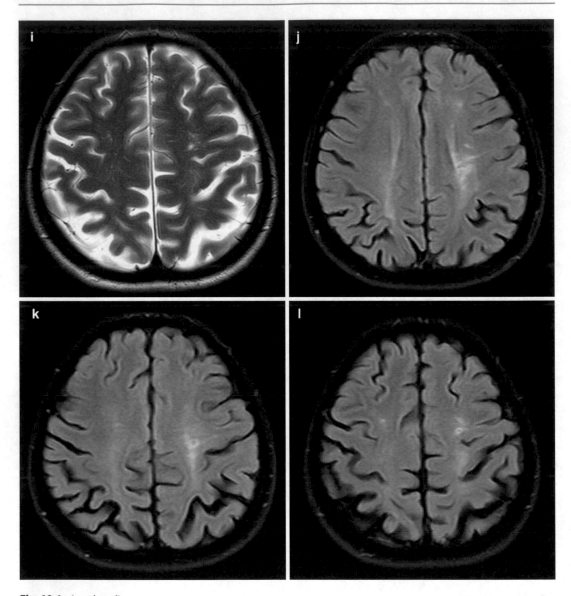

Fig. 12.1 (continued)

On hospital discharge antiphospholipid syndrome, triple positive, with elements of systemic lupus erythematosus (SLE), was diagnosed, and specific therapy, warfarin and methylprednisolone, was introduced. Six months after chloroquine phosphate was introduced in therapy, while warfarin and methylprednisolone doses were corrected. Follow-up brain MRI performed in June 2020 did not reveal difference of chronic vascular lesions in comparison to MRI from 2019, while MRA of cerebral arteries was unremarkable (Fig. 12.2).

12.1 Antiphospholipid Syndrome in a Patient with Systemic Lupus Erythematosus Elements

Antiphospholipid syndrome (APS) is defined as clinical autoimmune syndrome in which at least one of the clinical criteria and one of the laboratory criteria defined by revised Sapporo criteria are present. Laboratory criteria include persistent presence (detected on two or more occasions on testing at least 12 weeks apart) of antiphospho-

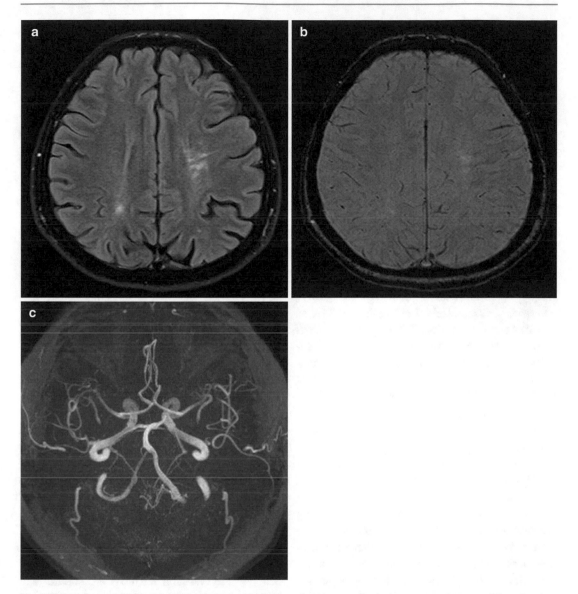

Fig. 12.2 Follow-up MRI of the brain performed in June 2020, non-contrast axial FLAIR (**a**), SWI (**b**) and 3D TOF MRA (**c**), in comparison to MRI, from 2019, there was no changes in number, size, shape and signal intensities of chronic vascular lesions reported as possibly related to antiphospholipid syndrome in comparison to MRI from 2019. MRA of cerebral arteries was unremarkable

lipid antibodies (aPLs): anticardiolipin antibodies of IgM or IgG isotype, anti-beta-2-glycoprotein 1 antibodies and lupus anticoagulant (LAC) in serum or plasma. Clinical criteria include acute arterial, venous or small vessel thrombosis in any tissue organ, and pregnancy morbidity including premature births, spontaneous abortions, and foetal death [1]. Non-thrombotic APS manifestations, which are not a part of Sapporo criteria, are thrombocytopenia, haemolytic anaemia, cardiac

valve disease (Libman–Sacks endocarditis), livedo reticularis and various neurologic manifestations including intractable headaches, migraines, seizures, chorea, transient ischemic attacks (TIAs) cerebrovascular accidents, amaurosis fugax, dementia, psychosis, depression, transverse myelitis and a multiple sclerosis-like disease.

The prevalence of APS positivity in apparently healthy individuals ranges from 1% to 5%

and increases with age, especially in older individuals with chronic diseases [2]. The mean age at the onset of the clinical manifestations of the disease is 31 years [3]. It affects females more frequently than males: female patients are often diagnosed through pregnancy loss.

This autoimmune syndrome can occur alone, as primary APS, or in the setting of other autoimmune conditions, in particular SLE, Sjögren's syndrome and rheumatoid arthritis, classified as secondary APS. Rarely, a life-threatening form of multiorgan thrombosis, known as catastrophic APS, can occur.

Huges originally described the syndrome in 1983 when he stressed the importance of cerebral features in these patients and accentuated the frequency of intractable headache or migraine, epilepsy, chorea, cerebral ischemia and TIA as the most common manifestation of the CNS involvement [4]. According to the Euro-Phospholipid Project Study Group, the cumulative prevalence of stroke and TIA in APS patients are 19.8 and 11.1%, respectively [3]. On the other hand, aPL antibodies may be detected in up to 13.5% of stroke patients, more often in young subjects [5].

Multiple effects of antiphospholipid antibodies exert alterations of the coagulation system at various levels in a prothrombotic manner explaining thrombotic manifestation of APS, including cerebral ischaemia [3]. Other neuropsychiatric manifestations of APS, like headache, movement disorders, seizures, cognitive dysfunction, multiple sclerosis-like disease, cannot be explained entirely by hypercoagulability. Those non-thrombotic manifestations have more complex causes like direct pathogenic effect of aPL antibodies which can bind to glial cells, myelin and neurons and disrupt their functions [6, 7]. Cerebral venous thrombosis is not a common manifestation of APS, because of a more selective vulnerability of the arterial system to thrombotic events [7].

Proposed pathogenic mechanism of epileptic seizures in APS is ischaemic damage to brain tissue, leading to formation of cortical epileptogenic foci. Antiphospholipid antibodies can impair GABA receptor activity and induce depolarization of synaptoneurosomes, disrupting neuronal function by acting on nerve terminals leading to epileptic seizure in structurally normal brain of a patient with APS [7, 8].

Chronic headache, including migraine, is a common finding in patients with APS [2] with an estimated prevalence of 20.2% [8]. Headache in APS is often untreatable, not responding to narcotics or analgesics and persisting for years before APS is diagnosed [6].

Most common CT and MRI findings in patients with APS are small hyperintense focal lesions in subcortical and periventricular white matter on T2WI and FLAIR, usually with normal T1-weighted signals and without contrast enhancement. Those lesions are often misdiagnosed as vasculitis, but they represent chronic, irreversible lesions in the setting of small vessel disease, therefore are not specific only for CNS involvement of APS.

More white matter hyperintensities than expected for patient age could be indicative of CNS involvement in a patient with anamnestic data suggestive of APS and positive aPL antibodies.

Other common imaging features of CNS involvement in APS are small cortical and lacunar infarcts, while large infarct in the territory of large cerebral arteries are less common [8]. The risk for recurrent stroke appears to be increased in APS patients, and multiple events can occur after the first cerebral ischaemic episode. Generally, the territory of the middle cerebral artery is more affected, but ischaemic events can occur in any vascular territory. We should take into consideration the fact that chronic multifocal vascular disease can produce multi-infarct dementia which can be difficult to differentiate from other kinds of dementia. Parietal lobe atrophy (postcentral gyrus) with relative sparing of frontal and temporal lobes could be seen in young patients with APS.

Preventing recurrent thrombosis in a patient with APS (secondary prevention) and preventing a first-episode thrombosis in a patient with aPL antibodies (primary prevention) using a non-anticoagulant agent that reduces thrombotic risk without increasing bleeding risk is the essence of therapy in APS [9].

With the exception of anticoagulation, there is no standard therapy for APS. The three stand-bys—aspirin, heparin and warfarin—remain the cornerstone of treatment.

Hydroxychloroquine (HCQ) is an antimalarial drug with anti-inflammatory and immunomodulatory properties that also blocks platelet aggregation and adhesion and improves cholesterol profiles. In their paper, Wang and Lim recommended it in patients with SLE and persistently positive aPL antibodies for the primary prevention of thrombosis. In patients without SLE but persistently positive aPL antibodies, they did not recommend HCQ in routine use of primary prevention of thrombosis [9].

EULA recommendations for the management of APS in adults published in 2019 define risk stratification in aPL-positive individuals, general measures for aPL-positive individuals and patient education and counselling on treatment adherence, and provide guidelines for specific therapy [10].

After diagnostic work-up in the hospital, the patient was diagnosed with antiphospholipid syndrome with SLE elements. She had a triple-positive antiphospholipid antibody profile that is defined as two positive serum IgG aPL antibodies along with one positive functional plasma lupus anticoagulant test result [11]. Such profile is associated with an increased risk for thrombosis, whereas patients with single-positive test results may have little to no increased risk [11].

According to anamnestic data and incomplete medical documentation, the patient had thrombotic and non-thrombotic APS symptoms over the years. She had headaches and well-controlled seizures as non-thrombotic symptoms, pregnancy pathology and brain MRI findings related to thrombotic events. With the first epileptic seizures, brain MRI was performed and white matter lesions were misunderstood as possibly related to vasculitis. Looking from our perspective backwards, it is possible to follow how this disease developed over the years with emerging typical symptoms and signs from seizures and pregnancy pathology, to headaches and arterial hypertension with newly confirmed renal pathology and positive specific aPL antibodies.

It is not easy for neuroradiologist to report small vessel vasculopathy due to APS on brain MRI if specific anamnestic and clinical data are not presented at the time of MRI study. Those lesions would probably be misdiagnosed for a small vessel vasculitis of unknown aetiology, and further diagnostic work-up would be recommended. Therefore, it is important that neurologist or immunologist provides neuroradiologist with proper anamnestic and clinical data or provides precise referral when recommending brain MRI. In the case, it would be easier for a neuroradiologist to differentiate such supratentorial white matter lesions as vasculitis or small vessel vasculopathy and direct diagnostic work-up towards possible specific autoimmune disorder.

In about a quarter of APSs, kidneys can be affected which can be presented as progressive kidney failure, proteinuria, sediment changes, renal infarction and, less commonly, acute renal failure. APS nephropathy is a vascular disease that affects glomerular tuft, interstitial vessels, and peritubular vessels; classic finding on histopathology is thrombotic microangiopathy. Kidney disease associates with aPL antibodies is not an inflammatory condition in contrast with lupus nephritis: it consists of arterial and venous renal thrombosis [12]. For cases with lupus nephritis, immunosuppressive therapy based on corticosteroid remains the mainstay of treatment. However, immunosuppression alone may be insufficient when antiphospholipid antibody syndrome and thrombotic microangiopathy are also present, and other treatment modalities including antiplatelet therapy, anticoagulation and plasma exchange are likely to be necessary, which was the case with introduced therapy for the patient [13].

References

1. Miyakis S, et al. International consensus statement on an update of the classification criteria for definite antiphospholipid syndrome (APS). J Thromb Haemost. 2006;4:295–306.
2. Petri M. Epidemiology of the antiphospholipid antibody syndrome. J Autoimmun. 2000;15:145–52.

3. Cervera R, et al. The euro-phospholipid project epidemiology of the antiphospholipid syndrome in Europe. Lupus. 2009;18:889–93.
4. Hughes GRV. Thrombosis, abortion, cerebral disease and the lupus anticoagulant. Br Med J. 1983;287:1088–9.
5. Andreoli L, et al. Estimated frequency of antiphospholipid antibodies in patients with pregnancy morbidity, stroke, myocardial infarction, and deep vein thrombosis: a critical review of the literature. Arthritis Care Res. 2013;65:1869–73.
6. Rodrigues CEM, et al. Neurological manifestations of antiphospholipid syndrome. Eur J Clin Investig. 2010;49(4):350–9.
7. Carecchio M, et al. Revisiting the molecular mechanism of neurological manifestations in antiphospholipid syndrome: beyond vascular damage. J Immunol Res. 2014;2014:239398. https://doi.org/10.1155/2014/239398.
8. Fleetwood T, et al. Antiphospholipid syndrome and the neurologist: from pathogenesis to therapy. Front Neurol. 2018;9:1001. https://doi.org/10.3389/fneur.2018.01001.
9. Wang TF, Lim W. What is the role of hydroxychloroquine in reducing thrombotic risk in patients with antiphospholipid antibodies? Haematol Am Soc Hematol Educ Program. 2016;2016(1):714–6.
10. Tektonidou M, et al. EULAR recommendations for the management of antiphospholipid syndrome in adults. Ann Rheum Dis. 2019;78:1296–304.
11. Froom P, et al. Triple positive antiphospholipid antibody profile in outpatients with tests for lupus anticoagulants. Clin Chem Lab Med. 2015;53(1):53–6.
12. Turrent-Carriles A, et al. Renal involvement in antiphospholipid syndrome. Front Immunol. 2018;9:1008. https://doi.org/10.3389/fimmu.2018.01008.
13. Sakamaki Y, et al. Renal thrombotic microangiopathy and antiphospholipid syndrome nephropathy in a patient with lupus nephritis. Nihon Jinzo Gakkai Shi. 2016;58(1):45–54.

Posterior Reversible Encephalopathy Syndrome (PRES): Holohemispheric Watershed Pattern

13

A 19-year-old male patient was transferred from a general hospital to our hospital due to additional diagnostic work-up of the chronic renal disease.

Five years ago, at the age of 15 years, he was diagnosed with chronic renal insufficiency: kidney biopsy revealed mesangial proliferative glomerulonephritis (MPGN). Such condition may occur in several renal diseases such as IgA nephropathy, lupus nephritis, post-infectious glomerulonephritis, which were quoted as a differential diagnosis. For 1 year, he was on recommended corticosteroid therapy: due to corticosteroid adverse effects, the patient self-initiated quitted therapy. For the past 3 years, he was not on corticosteroids, and he did not go for regular nephrologist check-ups or for renal function laboratory testing.

On admission to a general hospital, his general condition was seriously damaged, with high level of urea (73 mmol/L) and creatinine (2696 mmol/L), proteinuria, metabolic acidosis, anaemia, pleural and pericardial effusions. Haemodialysis was initiated, and when his general condition allowed, the patient was transferred to our hospital: on admission urea (32 mmol/L) and creatinine (1252 mmol/L) were increased, total protein levels, potassium and chlorides were within the normal range, sodium was slightly decreased. During his stay in our hospital, extensive diagnostic work-up was performed: systemic autoimmune disease or other systemic disease with renal manifestation (negative for Fabry disease) was not proven.

Therefore, nephrologists thought that in this case MPGN followed after tubulointerstitial nephritis.

During 2-weeks hospitalization, on a weekend in November 2018, neurologist on call asked for emergency brain CT due to the patient's first epileptic seizure. It was a grand mal seizure: generalised tonic clonic seizure with a loss of consciousness, arterial blood pressure was 195/120 mmHg. Clinician referrals for emergency brain CT were grand mal epileptic seizure, arterial hypertension and chronic renal disease.

General radiologist who was on call reported bilateral frontal and parietal cortical-subcortical hypodensities but did not specify to which condition those hypodensities could be attributed (Fig. 13.1).

MRI of the brain was performed 2 days after the epileptic seizure onset (Fig. 13.2): neuroradiologist reported radiomorphological changes consistent with holohemispheric watershed pattern of the posterior reversible encephalopathy syndrome (PRES). Those changes were in accordance with symptoms: grand mal epileptic seizure following increased arterial blood pressure in the setting of severe chronic renal insufficiency.

Afterwards haemodialysis was intensified, and antihypertensive medications and diazepam were introduced into therapy. Consequently, the patient was without epileptic seizures, arterial blood pressure was regulated, and follow-up MRI of the brain revealed significant vasogenic oedema regression (Fig. 13.3).

M. Špero, H. Vavro, *Neuroradiology - Images vs Symptoms*, https://doi.org/10.1007/978-3-030-69213-1_13

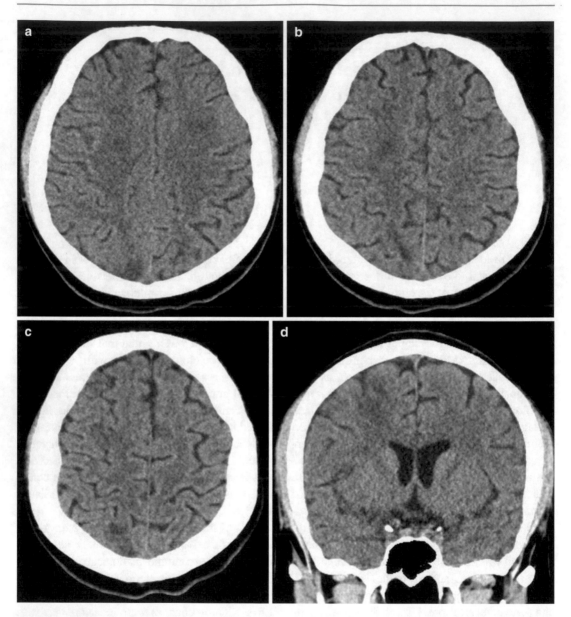

Fig. 13.1 Computed tomography of the brain, non-contrast, axial (**a–c**), coronal (**d**), sagittal (**e, f**) scans, revealed supratentorial bilateral, parasagittal subtle patchy, confluent, cortical-subcortical hypodensities in dorsal frontal and parietal lobes with narrowed adjacent sulci

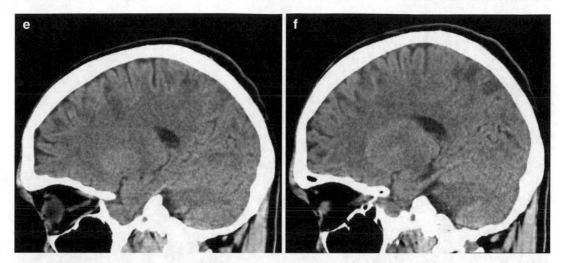

Fig. 13.1 (continued)

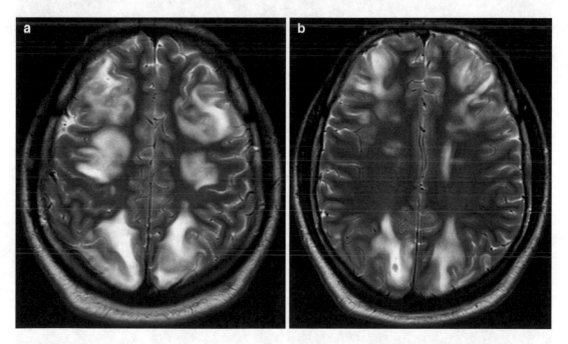

Fig. 13.2 Magnetic resonance imaging of the brain, non-contrast, axial T2WI (**a–c, g**), FLAIR FS (**d–f, j**), DWI (**h**), ADC (**k**), sagittal T1WI (**i, l**), performed 2 days after the epileptic seizure, revealed bilateral and symmetrical frontal, parietal and occipital lobes involvement with lesser temporal involvement. Subcortical white matter and, to a lesser extent, cortical grey matter demonstrated hypointense signal on T1WI, hypeintense signal on T2WI and FLAIR FS, hyperintense signal on DWI due T2 shine through with hyperintense signal on ADC maps, consistent with confluent vasogenic oedema. Involved gyri were slightly voluminous with narrow adjacent sulci

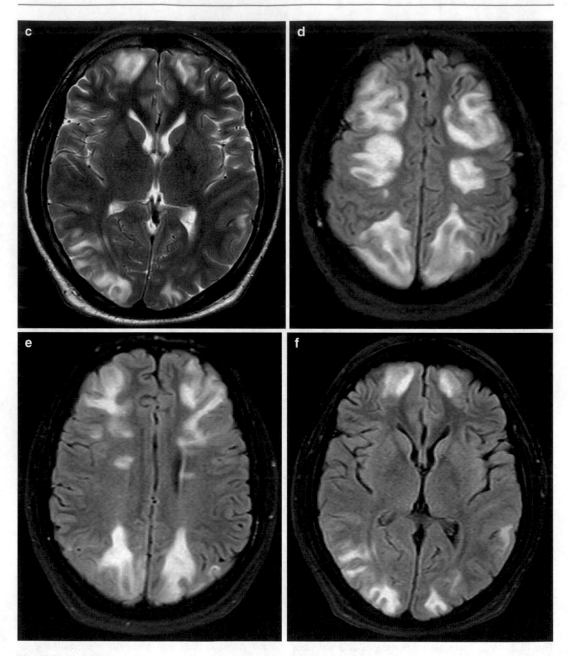

Fig. 13.2 (continued)

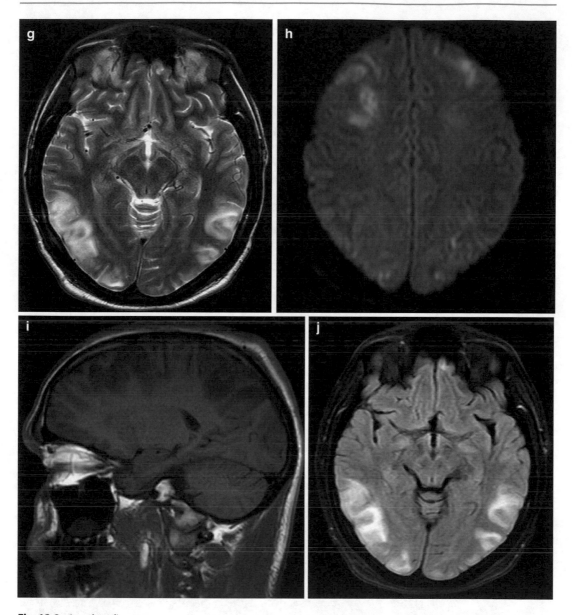

Fig. 13.2 (continued)

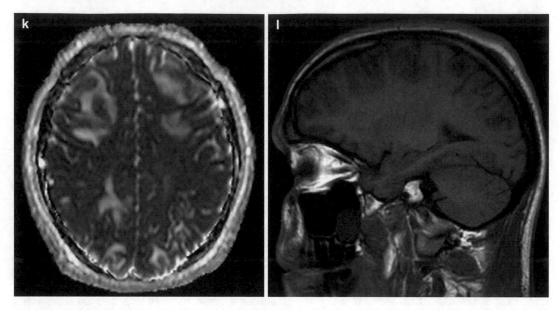

Fig. 13.2 (continued)

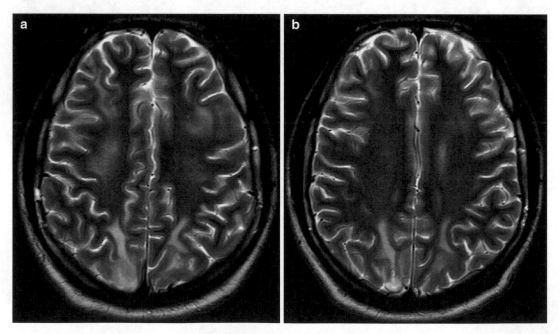

Fig. 13.3 Follow-up magnetic resonance imaging of the brain, axial T2WI (**a–c**) and FLAIR FS (**d–f**), performed 10 days after the first MRI, revealed significant vasogenic oedema regression. Involved gyri were not voluminous, and most of the adjacent sulci were not narrow any more, except in parietal lobes where changes showed moderate regressive dynamics as well

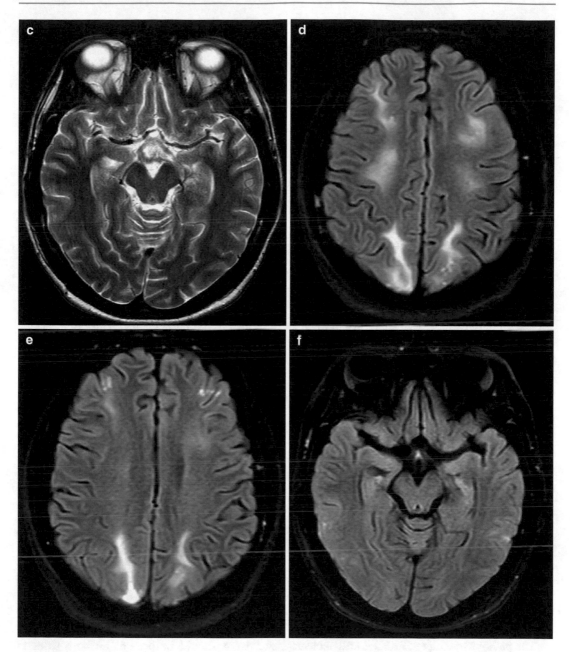

Fig. 13.3 (continued)

13.1 Posterior Reversible Encephalopathy Syndrome (PRES): Holohemispheric Watershed Pattern

Posterior reversible encephalopathy syndrome (PRES) is a clinical-radiological syndrome first described in 1996 by Hinchey and colleagues who named it reversible posterior leukoencephalopathy syndrome as it was considered that only white matter is involved in the syndrome [1]. Over the time, it became clear that the grey matter is involved as well, and the term posterior reversible encephalopathy syndrome was coined. This term is now widely accepted, but it is not entirely accurate because it is not exclusively posterior, nor is it always reversible [2].

Clinical manifestations, including headache, seizures, altered mental status and visual disturbances, may develop over several days or may be recognized only in the acute setting, both in children and in adults [3, 4]. Up to 75% of patients present with seizures: a single short grand mal seizure seems to be the most frequent seizure type. EEG in PRES does not seem to clearly mirror the propensity for generalized seizures. No clear correlation between MRI findings and EEG pathology exists [3].

Causes of PRES are diverse, but most cases of PRES occur due to acute elevation of blood pressure above the upper limit of cerebral blood flow autoregulation. Besides acute hypertension, PRES has been recognized in an increasing number of medical conditions, including preeclampsia/eclampsia, acute or chronic renal diseases, use of immunosuppressive drugs, chemotherapy, sepsis and collagen vascular disease [5].

The pathophysiology of PRES is still unclear: four hypotheses that try to explain it have been proposed till now. The first theory describes severe hypertension which exceeds the natural autoregulatory limits of the brain (150–160 mm Hg), with resultant injury to the capillary bed, fluid egress, and resultant vasogenic oedema. A competing theory describes the development of vasoconstriction due to autoregulatory compensation of severe hypertension leading to reduced brain perfusion, ischemia, and the development

of vasogenic oedema. Immune system activation with a resultant cascade which induces endothelial dysfunction and fluid leakage is a third theory attempting to explain the development of PRES [2, 6–8].

Largeau et al. have recently published a theory that arginine vasopressin (AVP) hypersecretion in different clinical conditions associated with the development of PRES, or AVP receptor density results in the activation of vasopressin V1a with associated cerebral vasoconstriction, endothelial dysfunction and cerebral ischaemia with resultant cytotoxic oedema. This may then lead to increased endothelial permeability and subsequent vasogenic oedema [9].

The combination of suggestive clinical manifestations and recognition of the characteristic imaging findings by radiologists is the key to diagnose this syndrome: PRES has both classic and atypical imaging features. In doubtful cases, the clinical and radiological improvement that occur once appropriate treatment is given confirms the diagnosis.

Due to syndrome clinical manifestations and availability of the imaging method, brain CT is the most commonly obtained screening procedure. MRI is superior to CT for the diagnosis of PRES and is the key investigation for the diagnosis and follow-up of this condition.

The classic imaging findings of PRES is focal or confluent vasogenic oedema involving subcortical white matter and often cortical grey matter of the parietal and occipital lobes. Frontal lobes (75–77%), temporal region (<65%) and cerebellum (50–55%) are additionally involved [7]. The distribution of vasogenic oedema is mainly symmetrical (71%), could be asymmetric, but it should be present on both sides in order to fulfil the diagnostic criteria for diagnosing PRES. Despite this, unilateral distributions of vasogenic oedema in PRES have been reported (Fig. 13.4). The predilection for the posterior brain is thought to be a result of the better-developed sympathetic regulation in the anterior circulation, with the posterior circulation more susceptible to impaired autoregulation and vasogenic oedema in the setting of hypertension.

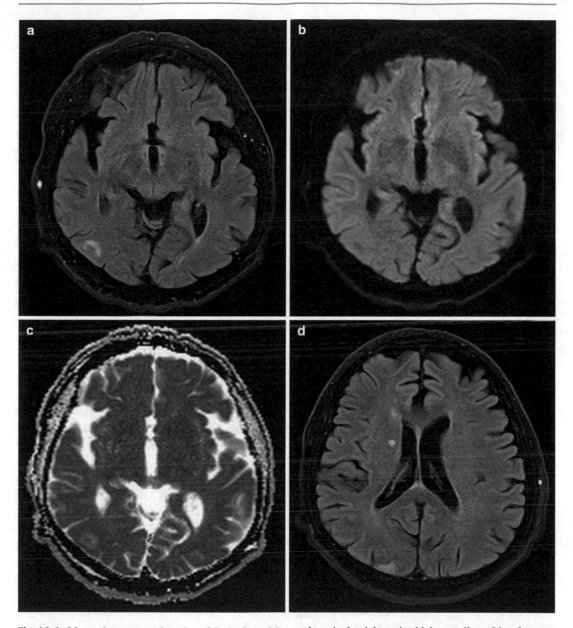

Fig. 13.4 Magnetic resonance imaging of the brain, axial FLAIR FS (**a**, **d**), DWI (**b**, **e**), ADC (**c**, **f**): patchy vasogenic oedema involving subcortical white matter in the right occipital lobe, and cortical-subcortical vasogenic oedema in the right parietal lobe—unilateral involvement in PRES (78-year-old male patient, acute hypertension). Vasogenic oedema is isointense on DWI and hyperintense on ADC—T2 washout

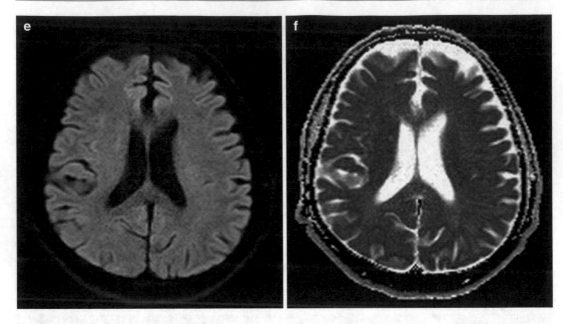

Fig. 13.4 (continued)

CT findings are often normal or nonspecific. Subtle patchy cortical/subcortical hypodensities on CT in a suggestive topographic distribution should raise suspicion of PRES. The typical vasogenic oedema encountered in the setting of PRES is best demonstrated with T2W and FLAIR sequences on MRI and is hypointense on corresponding T1WI. DWI usually confirms the vasogenic nature of this oedema with the absence of restricted diffusion. ADC values in areas of abnormal T2 signal intensity are typically elevated consistent with highly mobile water in areas of vasogenic oedema in PRES. These areas may appear hyperintense, hypointense, or isointense on DWI, depending on the amount of the T2 "shine-through" effect [7, 8, 10, 11]. The majority of lesions appear hypointense or isointense on DWI which is called T2 washout: isointense lesions on DWI result from a perfect balance of T2 effects and increased water diffusibility, whereas hypointense lesions on DWI have higher ADC values, which are not balanced by T2 effects (Fig. 13.4).

Intravenous contrast administration is not indicated to diagnose PRES but may be useful to exclude other clinical considerations. No enhancement or a slight leptomeningeal or gyral cortical enhancement is observed. Contrast enhancement is reported in a variable incidence, ranking from 23% to 43% and occurs secondary to the breakdown of the blood–brain barrier.

While variations exist in the most commonly encountered patterns of oedema distribution, Bartynski et al. described four lesion distribution patterns [4]. Holohemispheric watershed pattern (Fig. 13.2) is characterized by frontal, parietal and occipital lobe involvement with lesser temporal involvement consistent with watershed zones between the anterior and posterior cerebral arteries, on the one hand, and the middle cerebral artery, on the other. Bilateral vasogenic oedema involving the superior frontal sulcus area along the superior frontal sulci with varying degrees of parietal and occipital abnormalities defines superior frontal sulcus pattern. Dominant parietal-occipital pattern (Fig. 13.5) predominantly involves posterior part of the parietal and occipital lobes and was previously thought to be typical PRES [1–4, 11].

The fourth pattern is partial or asymmetric expression of primary patterns. In partial form, the frontal lobes are involved bilaterally, while parietal or occipital lobes are spared, while in asymmetric form there is unilateral absence of oedema in parietal or occipital lobes. In the partial and asymmetric forms, there is both absence of involvement of either the parietal or the occipital lobes and asymmetrical affection of the involved lobe [1–4, 11].

Involvement of the frontal lobes, cerebellum, basal ganglia and brainstem characterize atypical PRES which is not uncommon [12]. Knowledge of the different presentations of PRES is important, as atypical imaging findings should not

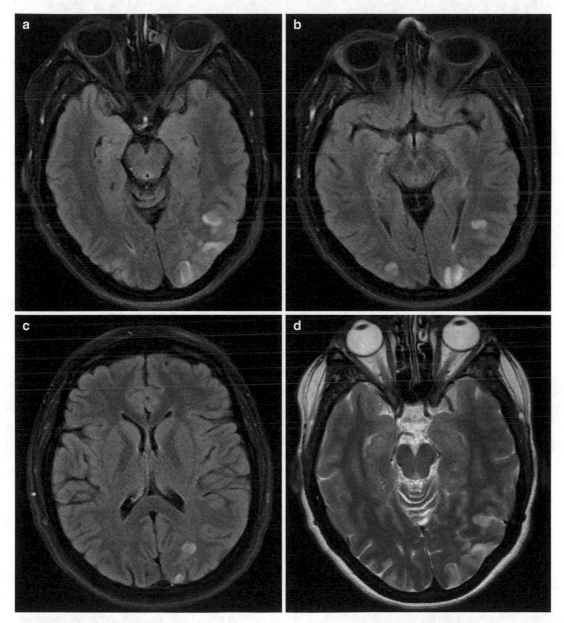

Fig. 13.5 Magnetic resonance of the brain, axial FLAIR FS (**a–c**) and T2WI (**d–f**), dominant parieto-occipital pattern of PRES: asymmetric patchy cortical-subcortical vasogenic oedema involving both occipital lobes and left parietal lobe (32-year-old female patient, 37 weeks pregnant, first grand mal epileptic seizure, arterial blood pressure 160/110 mmHg)

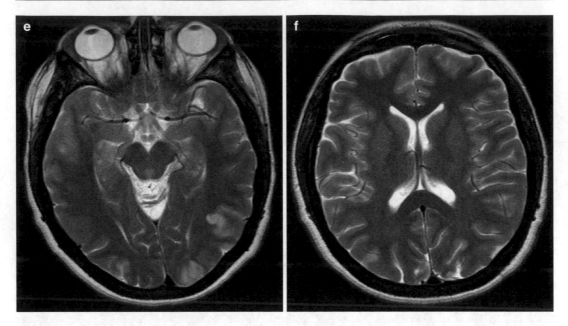

Fig. 13.5 (continued)

dissuade a diagnosis of PRES in the correct clinical context [12–14].

Intracranial haemorrhage is known to occur in PRES in approximately 15% to 65% of cases. The mechanism of haemorrhage in PRES may be secondary to pial vessel rupture in the setting of severe hypertension or reperfusion injury in the setting of vasoconstriction. Three different types of haemorrhage are identified: multifocal micro-haemorrhage (<5 mm), subarachnoid haemorrhage in cortical sulci or focal intraparenchymal haematomas. The risk seems to be greater in patients who have undergone allogeneic bone marrow transplants or organ transplants, as well as in patients taking anticoagulants [11].

There are cases of PRES that may be complicated by the development of cytotoxic oedema as indicated by diffusion restriction. Some cases may show reversibility of diffusion restriction similar to findings seen in patients with transient cerebral ischaemia, venous ischaemia/infarction, and vasospasm following subarachnoid haemorrhage although restriction often progresses to frank infarction with encephalomalacia identified on follow-up.

Focal or diffuse vasoconstriction, vasodilation or a 'string-of-beads' appearance most com-monly observed in the second- and third-order branches and frequently associated with regions of vasogenic oedema are reported in PRES at DSA. Such vessel irregularities can also be seen on CT or MR angiography. These findings may be confused for other diagnoses, such as vaso-spasm or vasculitis [3].

In PRES, MRS may show a reduced NAA peak. The presence of a lactate peak indicates cerebral infarction. Perfusion imaging shows a reduction in relative cerebral blood volume and cerebral blood flow in PRES, which supports the autoregulatory arterial vasoconstriction hypothe-sis leading to cerebral hypoperfusion, develop-ment of vasogenic oedema followed by cerebral ischaemia [14].

Differential diagnoses for imaging findings of PRES are mainly based on the distribution of the lesions. Important differential diagnoses are basi-lar top syndrome, venous infarction, trauma, vas-culitis, encephalitis and demyelinating disorders.

PRES must be diagnosed early and investiga-tions must be performed to identify the causative factors. Symptomatic treatment should be given immediately and the causative factors corrected without delay.

The syndrome is reversible if adequately treated. The patient very often makes good clinical progress with clinical signs improving relatively quickly. Imaging findings may take days or weeks to completely regress following initiation of treatment [15]. If treatment is not promptly initiated, PRES may progress to haemorrhage or infarction which are associated with poor prognosis, or even coma and death.

In case of our patient, the main cause of hypertension was chronic renal failure due to untreated MPGN probably after tubulointerstitial nephritis. Clinical manifestations of grand mal epileptic seizure and acute hypertension in the setting of chronic renal failure, and CT findings of bilateral, parasagittal patchy cortical-subcortical hypodensities in dorsal frontal and parietal lobes should have alerted suspicion of PRES with general radiologist who was on call during the weekend and had to give the report. I am sure experienced neuroradiologist would have not missed to report those hypodensities could be consistent with PRES. MRI of the brain was performed less than 48 h after the brain CT and revealed typical holohemispheric watershed pattern of PRES: in comparison to CT, imaging findings have significantly progressed during less than 48 h. Fortunately the patient's condition did not worsen during that time and epileptic seizure did not recur due to diazepam therapy. After the MRI, antihypertensive medications were introduced into therapy and arterial blood pressure was regulated. Follow-up MRI of the brain revealed significant vasogenic oedema regression.

Once again I would like to emphasize how important is that neuroradiologist reports CT and MRI of the brain and spine. In cases when neuroradiologist is not available and general radiologist has to report those, it is important that experienced neuroradiologist is consulted later for each difficult or doubtful case and revise reports if necessary. Therefore, further necessary diagnostic work-up and treatment would not be delayed.

References

1. Hinchey J, et al. A reversible posterior leukoencephalopathy syndrome. N Engl J Med. 1996;334:494–500.
2. Shankar J, Banfield J. Posterior reversible encephalopathy syndrome: a review. Can Assoc Radiol J. 2016;68(2):147–53.
3. Kastrup O, et al. Posterior reversible encephalopathy syndrome (PRES): electroencephalographic findings and seizure patterns. J Neurol. 2012;259:1383–9.
4. Bartynski WS. Posterior reversible encephalopathy syndrome, part 1: fundamental imaging and clinical features. AJNR Am J Neuroradiol. 2008;29(6):1036–42.
5. Saad AF, et al. Imaging of the atypical and complicated posterior reversible encephalopathy syndrome. Front Neurol. 2019;10:964.
6. Sudulagunta SR, et al. Posterior reversible encephalopathy syndrome (PRES). Oxf Med Case Reports. 2017;4:43–6.
7. Hugonnet E, et al. Posterior reversible encephalopathy syndrome (PRES): features on CT and MR imaging. Diagn Interv Imaging. 2013;94:45–52.
8. Siebert E, et al. Clinical and radiological spectrum of posterior reversible encephalopathy syndrome: does age make a difference? – a retrospective comparison between adult and pediatric patients. PLoS One. 2014;9(12):e115073.
9. Largeau B, et al. Arginine vasopressin and posterior reversible encephalopathy syndrome pathophysiology: the missing link? Mol Neurobiol. 2019;56:6792–806.
10. Abdul-Hameed AQI, et al. MRI features of posterior reversible encephalopathy syndrome. Egypt J Hosp Med. 2017;68(2):1229–35.
11. Ollivier M, et al. Neuroimaging features in posterior reversible encephalopathy syndrome: a pictorial review. J Neurol Sci. 2016;373:188–200. https://doi.org/10.1016/j.jns.2016.12.007.
12. McKinney AM, et al. Posterior reversible encephalopathy syndrome: incidence of atypical regions of involvment and imaging findings. AJR. 2007;189:904–12.
13. Stevens CJ, Heran MKS. The many faces of posterior reversible encephalopathy syndrome. Br J Radiol. 2012;85:1566–75.
14. Raman R, et al. Various imaging manifestations of posterior reversible encephalopathy syndrome (PRES) on magnetic resonance imaging (MRI). Pol J Radiol. 2017;82:64–70.
15. Legriel S, et al. Understanding posterior reversible encephalopathy syndrome. In: Vincent JL, editor. Annual update in intensive care and emergency medicine 2011. Annual update in intensive care and emergency medicine 2011, vol. 1. Berlin, Heidelberg: Springer; 2011.

Thrombotic Thrombocytopenic Purpura (TTP) and Haemolytic-Uremic Syndrome (HUS)

14

After what had seemed to be a simple urinary infection, this previously healthy 38-year-old woman developed thrombocytopenia; several months after that, she experienced visual field disturbances and facial paresthesia. Brain MRI reported microangiopathic parenchymal changes. A complete haematological work-up was undertaken, proving anaemia and very low ADAMTS13 enzyme activity with antibodies to it, consistent with TTP. Plasma exchange and corticosteroid therapy were started, but there were complications associated with catheter placement in terms of right leg deep venous thrombosis and hematothorax. Since therapy which also included vincristine and azathioprine did not give adequate results over several months, splenectomy was performed and plasma exchange was continued; thrombocytopenia started to improve and the platelet number was normal on the day of discharge from the hospital. However, she had to be readmitted 10 days later as platelet number started to decrease rapidly. Several days later, at the hospital, she had an epileptic seizure with fever and hypotension. Her platelet count remained stable, but signs of acute renal failure occurred. Urgent head CT was unremarkable:

Plasma exchange therapy had been continued, but 6 days later the patient developed a grand mal seizure with subsequent coma. Her platelet count plunged from 90×10^9/L to 67×10^9/L in a period of 24 h. Another urgent head CT was done, showing a large intracerebral haematoma (Fig. 14.1).

The patient had undergone an urgent neurosurgical brain decompression by a catheter placed in the brain ventricular system, but soon after that there was occlusion of the catheter by a thrombus which was removed by a neurosurgeon. Still, the patient remained out of contact, with unreactive pupils. A follow-up brain CT exam was called for, which demonstrated further worsening of the intracranial status (Fig. 14.2c).

Unfortunately, 2 days later, despite all the procedures and efforts, a hemodynamic collapse occurred which led to a fatal outcome.

14.1 Thrombotic Thrombocytopenic Purpura (TTP) and Haemolytic-Uremic Syndrome (HUS)

TTP and HUS are closely related, uncommon disorders characterized by microangiopathic haemolytic anaemia (MAHA) and thrombocytopenia [1]. Both the entities belong to a group of thrombotic microangiopathies (TMA), disorders characterized by microangiopathic haemolytic anaemia, thrombocytopenia and microthrombi, leading to ischaemic tissue injury. Incidence of TTP is between 1 and 13 cases per million, with 2:1 female to male predominance. In most cases, it occurs in people older than 40 years, but congenital forms may present in childhood. If untreated, mortality reaches 90%, whereas with

M. Špero, H. Vavro, *Neuroradiology - Images vs Symptoms*, https://doi.org/10.1007/978-3-030-69213-1_14

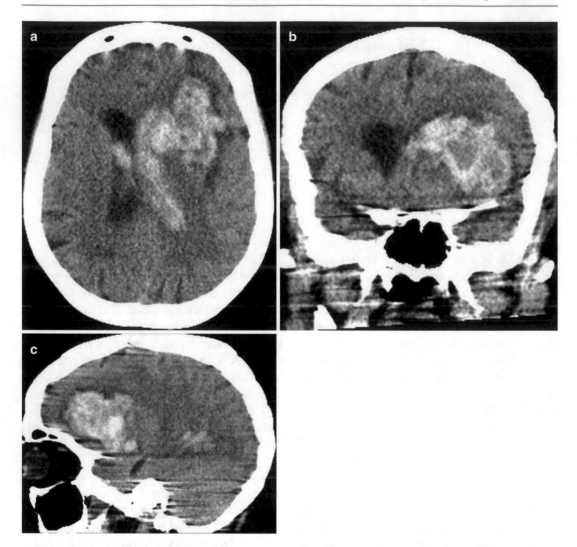

Fig. 14.1 Non-contrast CT exam of the brain. Axial (**a**), coronal (**b**) and sagittal (**c**) reformats. A large intracerebral haematoma (ICH) in the left frontal lobe with direct extension into the left ventricle. There is a rim of perifocal vasogenic oedema and a mild midline shift to the right

proper treatment it is fatal in 10–20%. Relapse occurs in up to 36% of patients [2].

Classical TTP should include haemolytic anaemia, thrombocytopenia, neurological symptoms, renal involvement and fever, but in practice only rare patients present with all five manifestations. In HUS, renal deficiency is the main clinical sign, it presents with MAHA and thrombocytopenia and often begins with diarrhoea [1]. TTP is caused by autoantibodies against the von Willebrand factor (VWF)-cleaving metalloprotease ADAMTS13, hence the

ultra large multimers of von Willebrand factor in the plasma of TTP patients [1]. Even if the auto-antibodies against ADAMTS13 are not detected, TTP may be confirmed if there is severe (<10 IU/dL) deficiency of ADAMTS13 in the plasma and MAHA and thrombocytopenia are diagnosed, and interfering conditions like infection, hematopoietic progenitor cell transplant (HPCT) and disseminated intravascular coagulation (DIC) are excluded. Normal to only moderately reduced (>20 IU/dL), ADAMTS13 plasma activity suggests atypical HUS (aHUS), especially with

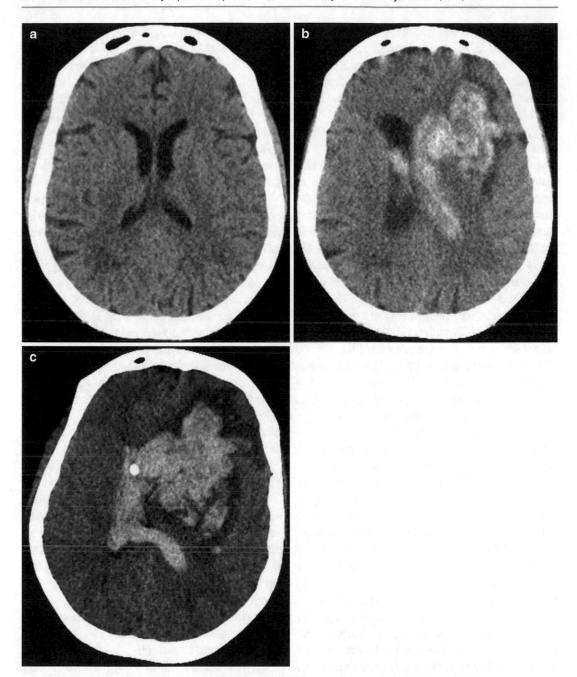

Fig. 14.2 Comparison of axial brain CT scans over time: after initial seizure (**a**); 6 days later, after the second, grand mal seizure (**b**); follow-up within the first 18 h after intraventricular catheter placement (**c**). There is marked worsening in (**c**), with ICH, oedema and midline shift progression. Note the hyperdense catheter in the anterior horn of the right lateral ventricle in (**c**)

predominant renal injury, or other types of thrombotic microangiopathy [2]. Most cases represent idiopathic TTP with sporadic HUS characterized by microvascular, platelet-rich angiopathy, also seen in HIV patients. In smaller percentage of cases, in which TTP-HUS is associated with malignancy and chemotherapy, the micro- and macrovascular thrombi are mainly composed of fibrin [1]. An acute episode of TTP may be triggered by infection, pregnancy, certain medications (clopidogrel, ticlopidine), complement and neutrophil activation and the release of human neutrophil peptides, extracellular DNA and histones [3].

Typical HUS (90% of cases) occurs after a diarrheal illness caused by *Escherichia coli* which produces Shiga toxin and is generally food-borne. Atypical HUS is very rare and is associated with excess activation or dysregulation of the alternate pathway of complement; it is mostly genetic, rarely acquired or idiopathic. Acute renal failure is featured in HUS but relatively rare in TTP, while MAHA, thrombocytopenia and diarrheal onset make it similar to TTP. Neurological complications such as stroke, seizure, coma and hemiparesis affect no more than 50% of HUS patients, but are among the main causes of their acute mortality [4].

Differential diagnoses of MAHA with thrombocytopenia which do not fall under TMA group include HELLP syndrome, severe hypertension, severe sepsis and DIC, malignant disease, autoimmune process, mechanical causes such as implanted shunts and valves, paroxysmal nocturnal haemoglobinuria and transplant patients.

TTP affects CNS more than any other organ or system as CNS is very sensitive to oxygen depletion caused by thrombi forming in arterioles and capillaries. Neurological presentation is a feature of more than 50% of episodes [2, 5]. Neurologic symptoms include headache, focal neurologic deficits, seizures, confusion and vertigo, eventually even coma and death. Other frequent symptoms are weakness, fever, arthralgia, myalgia, jaundice, nausea, vomiting, diarrhoea and abdominal pain [6]. Frequently, the presentation of TTP is indolent, symptoms may be fluctuating, taking days or weeks of malaise until the diagnosis is established in an ambulatory setting [2].

On imaging, brain CT and MRI may be normal, although brain MRI may demonstrate hyperintense foci in T2WI. Normal CT findings suggest likely full clinical recovery [5], even in cases with marked clinical findings. Approximately 25% of patients have changes visible on brain CT, with PRES (posterior reversible encephalop-

athy syndrome) making one half of these abnormalities, consisting of vasogenic oedema in parietal and occipital regions (for more information on PRES, see Chap. 13 of this book). Majority of these imaging abnormalities are reversed by treatment [7]. As vasospasm is associated with PRES, it may also be involved in infarctions and haemorrhages (ICH) in TTP. ICH may develop on account on severe hypertension and low platelet count [8].

Treatment of choice for acquired TTP is therapeutic plasma exchange (TPE, plasmapheresis), due to antibodies against ADAMTS13. Plasma infusions may serve as a short-term measure only. Fresh frozen plasma is usually applied. Doses vary from 5 ml/kg every 2 weeks for prophylactic use to 10 ml/kg once a week or every 2 weeks for treating acute TTP. High-dose steroids are also used (1 mg/kg) [2]. Physicians usually refrain from giving platelet transfusions, as there are already platelet-rich thrombi in the vessels; this procedure should be reserved for patients with overt bleeding and patients with severe thrombocytopenia undergoing invasive procedures [3, 5]. Gene therapy is under development.

Acute stroke therapy: according to both the European Stroke Organization (ESO) and the American Heart Association (AHA) guidelines and the drug insert, platelet count under $100 \times 10^9/L$ is a contraindication for giving IV rtPA for stroke, although by AHA it is not necessary to await platelet counts prior to administering IV rtPA unless there is a suspected thrombocytopenia [9].

Approximately 0.5–0.8% of patients treated for stroke are thrombocytopenic [10, 11], which is usually established after applying therapy. Thus, the overall number of patients is very small, and there are no dedicated studies on this topic, especially in patients with severe thrombocytopenia (platelet count of less than $40 \times 10^9/L$). However, the outcomes were not different compared to patients with normal platelet counts. In cases of full-dose thrombolytic therapy applied in known [12] and unknown [13] TTP thrombocytopenia cases with platelet count of less than $30 \times 10^9/L$, as well as in a case where drug application was aborted as soon as the (low) platelet count was available [14], there was no ICH; in the first two cases, TPE was proven to be beneficial when applied after rTPA (24 hours in the first case, 48 h in the second case), and the symptoms have resolved.

Mechanical thrombectomy could be a safer alternative to rTPA for stroke therapy in cases with significant thrombocytopenia, but the number of reported cases is still too low to recommend it as a standard [11].

References

1. Levandovsky M, et al. Thrombotic thrombocytopenic purpura-hemolytic uremic syndrome (TTP-HUS): a 24-year clinical experience with 178 patients. J Hematol Oncol. 2008;1:23. https://doi.org/10.1186/1756-8722-1-23.
2. Stanley M, Michalski JM. Thrombotic Thrombocytopenic Purpura (TTP) [Updated 2020 Jun 11]. In: StatPearls [Internet]. Treasure Island, FL: StatPearls Publishing; 2020. Available from: https://www.ncbi.nlm.nih.gov/books/NBK430721/.
3. Saha M, et al. Thrombotic thrombocytopenic purpura: pathogenesis, diagnosis and potential novel therapeutics. J Thromb Haemost. 2017;15(10):1889–900. https://doi.org/10.1111/jth.13764.
4. Hosaka T, et al. Hemolytic uremic syndrome-associated encephalopathy successfully treated with corticosteroids. Int Med (Tokyo, Japan). 2017;56(21):2937–41. https://doi.org/10.2169/internalmedicine.8341-16.
5. Kelly FE, et al. Coma in thrombotic thrombocytopenic purpura. J Neurol Neurosurg Psychiatry. 1999;66(5):689–90. https://doi.org/10.1136/jnnp.66.5.689.
6. Aksay E, et al. Thrombotic thrombocytopenic purpura mimicking acute ischemic stroke. Emerg Med J. 2006;23(9):e51. https://doi.org/10.1136/emj.2006.036327.
7. D'Aprile P, et al. Thrombotic thrombocytopenic purpura: MR demonstration of reversible brain abnormalities. AJNR Am J Neuroradiol. 1994;15(1):19–20.
8. Duncan IC. Cerebral vasospasm and intracerebral haemorrhage in a case of pregnancy-related thrombotic thrombocytopoenic purpura/haemolytic uraemic syndrome. Interv Neuroradiol. 2005;11(2):173–8. https://doi.org/10.1177/159101990501100209.
9. Fugate JE, Rabinstein AA. Absolute and relative contraindications to iv rt-pa for acute ischemic stroke. Neurohospitalist. 2015;5(3):110–21. https://doi.org/10.1177/1941874415578532.
10. Breuer L, et al. Waiting for platelet counts causes unsubstantiated delay of thrombolysis therapy. Eur Neurol. 2013;69(5):317–20. https://doi.org/10.1159/000345702.
11. Onder H, et al. Acute middle cerebral artery occlusion treated by thrombectomy in a patient with myelodysplastic syndrome and severe thrombocytopenia. J Vasc Interv Neurol. 2015;8(4):22–6.
12. Boattini M, Procaccianti G. Stroke due to typical thrombotic thrombocytopenic purpura treated successfully with intravenous thrombolysis and therapeutic plasma exchange. BMJ Case Rep. 2013;2013:bcr2012008426. https://doi.org/10.1136/bcr-2012-008426.
13. Badugu P, Idowu M. Atypical thrombotic thrombocytopenic purpura presenting as stroke. Case Rep Hematol. 2019;2019(7425320):14. https://doi.org/10.1155/2019/7425320.
14. Acır İ, Erdoğan HA, Yayla V, Tuşdemir N, Çabalar M. Incidental thrombotic thrombocytopenic purpura during acute ischemic stroke and thrombolytic treatment. J Stroke Cerebrovasc Dis. 2018;27(5):1417–9. https://doi.org/10.1016/j.jstrokecerebrovasdis.2017.10.032.

Citrobacter koseri Brain Abscess in Chronic Cocaine Addict

15

A 48-year-old male patient was admitted to the EHD due to intermittent twitches affecting right half of the face lasting for 5 days. Twitches were considered as partial seizures and were followed by right sided hemiparesis and motoric dysphasia lasting for 3 days.

The patient was a chronic drug addict. In the early phase of his addiction, he was using heroin intravenously. For the past several years, he was using cocaine intranasally, sniffing. For about 1.5 years before this episode, he was using high doses of cocaine: according to anamnestic data, 2 days before the admission, he took 10 g of cocaine. The patient also suffered from psycho-organic syndrome due to long-lasting drug addiction. On admission he was afebrile, C-reactive protein was elevated (38.6 mg/L), while the rest of the laboratory findings, including blood count, prothrombin time, urea, creatinine, electrolytes and liver function tests were normal. He was also tested for drugs and was positive for cocaine and benzodiazepines, and negative for amphetamine, meta-amphetamine, 3–4 methylenedioxymethamphetamine, morphine, opiates, methadone and tetrahydrocannabinol.

Brain CT was performed in the EHD and reported by interventional radiologist who was on call (Fig. 15.1).

Brain CT was performed without contrast media application because it was not possible to set up intravenous line at that time. Radiologist on call reported intra-axial expansile mass in the left frontal lobe suspected to be primary brain tumour (Fig. 15.1). Neurologist did not inform radiologist that the patient was a cocaine addict and the information was not entered into hospital information system at the time.

Furthermore, the patient was tested for HBV, HCV and HIV: he was negative for HCV and HIV, hepatitis B surface antigen (HbsAg) and antibody to hepatitis B core antigen (anti-HBc) were negative, while antibody to hepatitis B surface antigen (anti-HBs) was positive (5.26 IU/L), indicating either recovering from the past infection or the patient received hepatitis B vaccine.

Brain MRI was performed and reported by neuroradiologist 2 days after the brain CT (Fig. 15.2).

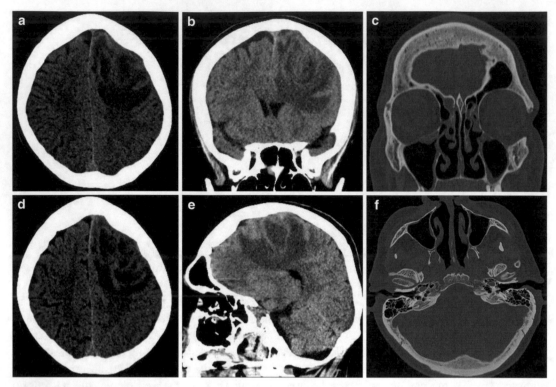

Fig. 15.1 Computed tomography of the brain, non-contrast, axial (**a**, **d**), coronal (**b**), sagittal (**e**) scans, bone window coronal (**c**), axial (**f**) scans, performed in the EHD revealed supratentorial intra-axial left frontal large expansile mass with perilesional oedema, reduced adjacent sulci and compressed frontal horn of the left lateral ventricle. Few nasal septal perforation, thinning of the middle and inferior turbinate and its mucosa, hard palate and paranasal sinuses walls were intact on bone window (**c**, **f**). There were no evidence of paranasal sinusitis or otomastoiditis

According to radiomorphological characteristics typical for pyogenic abscess, I reported mass was not a primary brain tumour, but pyogenic brain abscess.

The patient underwent left frontal trepanation and abscess content was drained. Samples of purulent content taken for microbiological analysis revealed *Citrobacter koseri* as microbiological pathogen. Follow-up CT revealed proper position of a drainage system. Antibiotic therapy was conducted with specific antibiotics according to antimicrobial susceptibility testing—he was treated with meropenem and vancomycin intravenously.

About after 3–4 weeks, the patient underwent left frontal craniotomy due to deterioration in mental state: purulent content was drained and the rest of the abscess cavities were removed completely. Final pathologist report was consistent with the brain abscess.

Specific antibiotic therapy was continued with meropenem intravenously. Conducted surgical and medicamentous treatment had favourable outcome.

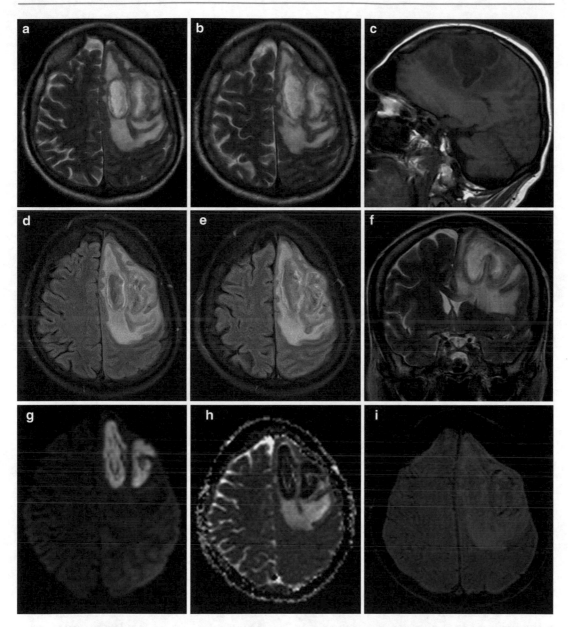

Fig. 15.2 Magnetic resonance of the brain, non-contrast axial T2WI (**a**, **d**) FLAIR FS (**b**, **e**) sagittal T1WI (**c**), coronal T2WI (**f**), axial DWI (**g**), ADC (**h**), SWI (**i**), post-contrast axial T1 MPRAGE (**j–l**), revealed pyogenic brain abscess in the left frontal lobe consisting of two connecting abscess cavities (**b**, **e**, **f**, **l**). Intra-axial left frontal mass showed "dual rim" sign of the capsule on T2WI/FLAIR and SWI, which was slightly hyperintense on non-contrast T1WI. On DWI mass demonstrated high signal centrally with hypointense signal and ADC representing true restricted diffusion. On axial post-contrast T1 MPRAGE smooth, complete rim of enhancement was noted

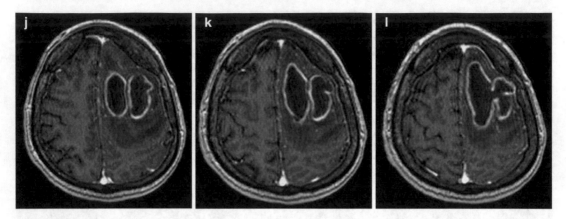

Fig. 15.2 (contiunued)

15.1 *Citrobacter koseri* Brain Abscess in Chronic Cocaine Addict

After cannabis, cocaine is the most frequently used illegal drug globally. It is a powerful nervous system stimulant often used as a recreational drug. Cocaine is presented in a form of cocaine hydrochloride, a fine white powder injected, inhaled or rubbed along the oral gum line, and in smokable form, crack cocaine, made by processing cocaine with sodium bicarbonate and water.

Brain abscess is a focal infection of the brain that begins as a localized area of cerebritis and develops into a collection of pus surrounded by a well-vascularized capsule.

Abscesses account for 1–2% of brain occupying space lesions in western countries and 8% in developing countries [1]. They are uniformly more common among males than females for unknown reasons and most commonly occurs during the first four decades of life, although all age groups may be affected. Early recognition and prompt treatment are essential for survival.

Pyogenic brain abscesses are not common, accounting for one third of all the cerebral abscesses. The most common identified causes of brain abscess include direct spread from local infections (sinusitis, otitis, mastoiditis), haematogenous dissemination from a distant source,

trauma and neurosurgical complication [2, 3]. Up to 30% of brain abscesses are reported as cryptogenic [2]. Additional predisposing factors include diabetes mellitus, alcoholism, intravenous drug abuse, pulmonary AVM, and immunosuppression. Pyogenic brain abscess is the most important secondary complication of heroin abuse following endocarditis due to non-sterile conditions associated with intravenous drug abuse, and *Staphylococcus aureus* is the most common pathogen [3].

Clinical features are different according to the location or mass effect of the abscess. Otomastoiditis causes abscess formation in the adjacent temporal lobe and cerebellum. Frontal and ethmoid sinusitis and odontogenic infection are frequently associated with the formation of frontal lobe abscess. Abscesses secondary to haematogenous seeding from a distant source are more typically multiple, near the grey–white junction, and usually in the distribution of the middle cerebral artery. Headache, nausea, emesis, fever, alteration in consciousness, seizures and motor weakness are the most common symptoms. These symptoms are more rapidly progressive with respect to tumoral lesions.

Pyogenic brain abscesses develop in response to a parenchymal infection with pyogenic bacteria, which begins as a localized area of cerebritis and evolves into a suppurative lesion surrounded by a well-vascularized fibrotic capsule [4]. Imaging features of a brain abscess depend on the stage at the time of imaging as well as the source of infection. Brain abscess development can be divided into four stages. The early cerebritis occurs from days 1–3 and is typified by neutrophil accumulation, tissue necrosis and oedema. The late cerebritis occurs from days 4–9 and is associated with a predominant macrophage and lymphocyte infiltrate. The capsule stage occurs from day 10 onward and is associated with the formation of a well-vascularized abscess wall, in effect sequestering the lesion and protecting the surrounding normal brain parenchyma from additional damage. Early capsule formation develops from days 10–13 and tends to be thinner on the medial or ventricular side of the abscess and prone to rupture in this direction. After day 14, late capsule formation develops, with gliotic, collagenous and granulation layers [1–3]. In addition to limiting the extent of infection, the immune response that is an essential part of abscess formation also destroys the surrounding normal brain tissue.

The majority of abscesses demonstrate considerable surrounding oedema secondary to mass effect. CT and MR imaging findings depend on the stage of the infection. In the earlier phases, a non-contrast CT scan may show only hypodense abnormalities with mass effect. In later phases, a complete peripheral ring may be seen revealing uniform ring enhancement on post-contrast CT scans [1, 2].

In the early phase, lesions revealed on MR images can have hypointense signal on T1WI and a hyperintense signal on T2WI, with patchy contrast enhancement on post-contrast T1WI. The typical MRI appearance of a pyogenic brain abscess is a ring-enhancing lesion with a rim that is isointense to hyperintense relative to white matter on non-contrast T1WI and hypointense on T2WI, surrounding a necrotic centre. Characteristic peripheral T1 and T2 signal shortening may be due to collagen, haemorrhage or free radicals. Content of the abscess cavity has low or intermediate signal intensity on T1WI, is hyperintense on T2WI (hypointense to CSF) and does not attenuate on FLAIR [4, 5].

Necrotic material in cerebral abscesses contains inflammatory cells, a matrix of proteins, cellular debris and bacteria in high-viscosity pus; all of these factors restrict water motion. Therefore, pyogenic brain abscess reveals restricted diffusion with characteristic hyperintensity on DWI and corresponding hypointensity on ADC.

Pyogenic brain abscess has a characteristic appearance of a concentric hypointense rim surrounding a hyperintense rim on T2WI/FLAIR and SWI which is called a "dual rim sign". It is found in the SWI due to its sensitivity to both paramagnetic and diamagnetic substances. The end products by macrophages of paramagnetic free radicals have been proposed to be responsible for the hypointense rim of fibrocollagenous capsule, which is usually smooth and complete, while granulation tissues line the inner part of the abscess capsule and are responsible for the hyperintense signal [2, 4, 5].

Abscesses tend to grow towards the white matter, away from the better-vascularized grey matter, with thinning of the medial wall due to relative hypovascularity in this region. This finding is thought to relate to the propensity of abscess to decompress into the ventricles in advanced stages of the disease.

MR spectroscopy has been shown to be specifically useful in differentiating between brain abscesses and other cystic lesions. Metabolic substances, such as succinate (2.4 ppm), acetate (1.9 ppm), alanine (1.5 ppm), amino acids (0.9 ppm), and lactate (1.3 ppm), can all be present in untreated bacterial abscesses on MR spectroscopy and are not present in glioblastoma [3].

The role of perfusion imaging, specifically the calculated rCBV, is an estimation of the angiogenesis. Enhancing rim in pyogenic brain abscess lacks neovascularization and histologically the microvascular density, and thus, it demonstrates low rCBV values [5].

It is important to differentiate pyogenic brain abscess from other ring-enhancing lesions with perifocal oedema, like glioblastoma or metastasis, to determine the indications and urgency of intervention and a suitable management plan. Advanced MRI techniques complement the role of conventional MRI in the differential diagnosis between these entities.

The clinical value of DWI lies in the ability to readily differentiate pyogenic brain abscess from necrotic brain tumour. Necrotic material in tumours contains cellular debris, serous fluid and fewer inflammatory cells; thus, water molecules have a greater freedom of motion. Most necrotic tumours reveal mildly increased diffusion with low-to-intermediate signal intensity on DWI and high ADC values in comparison to reduced diffusion and low ADCs in abscess [2, 5–7].

The dual rim sign has been reported to be the most specific feature in differentiating brain abscess from glioblastoma on SWI. The random deposition of haemorrhagic products in glioblastoma causes the presence of irregular and incomplete hypointense rim surrounding the necrotic centre. Pyogenic brain abscess, and not glioblastoma, has a characteristic appearance a "dual rim sign" [2, 4].

The degree of angiogenesis is associated with tumour aggressiveness. Enhancing rim in tumour contains viable tumour and thereby demonstrates an increased rCBV. Enhancing rim in a pyogenic brain abscess demonstrates lower rCBV values on PWI compared to glioblastoma.

In terms of CT and MR imaging features, our case is an example of typical pyogenic brain abscess with smooth, complete capsule hyperintense on non-contrast T1WI, revealing "dual rim" sign on T2WI/FLAIR and SWI, restricted diffusion in the centre and rim contrast enhancement on post-contrast T1WI. Circumstances in which the abscess developed and the specific causative agent were different.

Cocaine induces vascular CNS complications in the form of ischaemic stroke and intracranial haemorrhage. Pyogenic brain abscess is not typical complication of cocaine addiction. In a case of midfacial bone destruction due to chronic intranasal cocaine abuse and superimposed infection, route for its intracranial spread could be considered [8].

Brain CT performed in the EHD revealed intra-axial left frontal mass that resembled primary brain tumour/glioblastoma to interventional radiologist who was on call. It also revealed nasal septal perforation and thinning of the middle and inferior turbinate and its mucosa which are expected findings in chronic intranasal cocaine abuse. The radiologist on call missed those findings, and he was also not informed that the patient was cocaine addict. Those information would be helpful to radiologist to report CT findings in a different way and recommend brain MRI. If neuroradiologist would have reported this, CT nasal septal and turbinate changes would probably alert neuroradiologist to think about possible drug abuse and brain abscess, discuss that possibility with attending neurologist and recommend MRI.

Intranasal cocaine abuse induces vasoconstriction and focal ischaemia that might cause necrosis in the mucosae and surrounding tissues (cartilaginous and osseous) [9]. Therefore, frequent intranasal sniffing of cocaine hydrochloride powder may result in nasal septal perforation and destruction and may even progress to extensive paranasal destruction involving turbinate, paranasal sinus walls, cribriform plate, orbit and hard palate. Such conditions must be differentiated from aggressive neoplasia, inflammatory or infectious process.

Citrobacter koseri (CK), formerly known as *Citrobacter diversus*, is a gram-negative bacillus that belongs to the family Enterobacteriaceae. It colonizes gastrointestinal and urogenital tract of humans and is also present in soil and water [10, 11]. CK causes mostly meningitis and brain abscess in neonates and infants. It is responsible for 1.3% of cases of neonatal meningitis: brain abscess is seen in 76% of Citrobacter-related meningitis cases [10, 11]. Mechanisms that explain predilection of CK for infecting the central nervous system have not been clarified, although bacterial resistance to phagocytosis has been observed by Azrak et al. In addition, a particular 32 kDa protein in the external membrane of the bacteria has been identified; this seems to have meningeal tropism, as well as a tendency to produce abscesses and ventriculitis [11]. Brain abscess caused by *Citrobacter koseri* in an adult is extremely rare, and only three cases have been described in the literature [11–13]. How did *Citrobacter koseri* invade brain in case of this patient remains unknown. The patient was not immunocompromised patient, he did not have urinary infection.

Because of the rarity of the cases of adult brain abscess caused by *Citrobacter koseri* infection, the "gold standard" of treatment remains unknown. Although conservative treatment with antibiotics alone has been reported to be successful in the management of paediatric *Citrobacter koseri* brain abscesses, early aggressive surgical intervention followed by medical management is highly recommended, especially when encapsulated or multi-lobulated brain abscesses form. In general, *Citrobacter koseri* is usually resistant to ampicillin and has variable susceptibility to aminoglycosides. Despite the antibiotic susceptibility tests, third-generation cephalosporin, aminoglycosides or trimethoprim is the recommended antimicrobial agents [11].

References

1. Muccio CF, et al. Magnetic resonance features of pyogenic brain abscesses and differential diagnosis using morphological and functional imaging studies: a pictorial essay. J Neuroradiol. 2014;41:153–67.
2. Rath TJ, et al. Imaging of cerebritis, encephalitis, and brain abscess. Neuroimaging Clin N Am. 2012;22:585–607.
3. Erdogan E, Cansever T. Pyogenic brain abscess. Neurosurg Focus. 2008;24(6):2–10.
4. Antulov R, et al. Differentiation of pyogenic and fungal brain abscesses with susceptibility-weighted MR sequences. Neuroradiology. 2014;56(11):937–45.
5. Hakim A, et al. Pyogenic brain abscess with atypical features resembling glioblastoma in advanced MRI imaging. Radiol Case Rep. 2017;12:365–70.
6. Villanueva-Meyer J, Cha S. From shades of gray to microbiologic imaging: a historical review of brain abscess imaging. Radiographics. 2015;35:1555–62.
7. Cartes-Zumelzu FW, et al. Diffusion-weighted imaging in the assessment of brain abscesses therapy. AJNR Am J Neuroradiol. 2004;25:1310–7.
8. Ballage A, et al. Nasal septum perforation due to cocaine abuse. SAJ Case Rep. 2017;4:302–5.
9. Armstrong M Jr, et al. Nasal septal necrosis mimicking Wegener's granulomatosis in a cocaine abuser. Ear Nose Throat J. 1996;75(9):623–6.
10. Nunez Cuadros E, et al. Medical and neurosurgical management of Citrobacter koseri, a rare cause of neonatal meningitis. J Med Microbiol. 2014;63:144–7.
11. Liu HW, et al. Brain abscess caused by Citrobacter koseri infection in an adult. Neurosciences. 2015;20(2):170–2.
12. Booth LV, et al. Citrobacter diversus ventriculitis and brain abscesses in an adult. J Infect. 1993;26:207–9.
13. Lind CR, et al. Peritumoral Citrobacter koseri abscess associated with parasagittal meningioma. Neurosurgery. 2005;57:E814.

A 70-year-old man was examined in the ER department because of a sudden loss of consciousness followed by confusion. During the neurological examination and work-up, he experienced a seizure. He also demonstrated left-sided weakness. His medical history included surgery and irradiation for prostatic carcinoma and hypertension.

A CT exam of the brain was requested by a neurologist, particularly to check for intracranial space-occupying lesions (Fig. 16.1).

The work-up continued with an MRI of the brain (Fig. 16.2).

After the diagnosis of an intraventricular meningioma had been confirmed by MRI, the patient underwent surgery which was uneventful. Histopathology findings reported a WHO grade II meningioma.

Another patient, a 60-year-old man, had been lethargic and depressed, with cognitive impairment, forgetfulness and drowsiness in the month prior to being admitted to hospital. A few days prior to arrival to our facility, he became disoriented, agitated during the night, ataxic, did not recognize family members nor household items.

After a psychiatrical and neurological evaluation, he underwent a brain CT exam (Fig. 16.3a, b), followed by a brain MRI exam (Fig. 16.3c–f):

The patient underwent surgery which resulted in complete removal of the tumour.

Two days later, a postoperative MRI exam was performed (Fig. 16.4):

The histopathology confirmed the tumour was an atypical meningioma (WHO grade II).

16.1 Intraventricular Meningioma (IVM)

Primary intraventricular meningiomas make approximately 0.5–3% of all intracranial meningiomas [1] and therefore are very rare lesions. Still, they remain a neurosurgical challenge due to their size at the time of diagnosis, proximity to vital intraventricular structures and vascular supply which can be evaluated only after significant debulking [2]. Most are sited in the trigones of the lateral ventricles, left more often than right. They are more common in women (2.1:1 female-to-male ratio) [1] and peak at 30–60 years of age. Usually they are quite large at the time of diagnosis. Most commonly they present with raised intracranial pressure (70%), visual impairment (27%), dizziness (24%), motor deficits, sensory disturbances, cognitive and personality disturbances (10%) and gait ataxia [1]. Seizures, both

M. Špero, H. Vavro, *Neuroradiology - Images vs Symptoms*,
https://doi.org/10.1007/978-3-030-69213-1_16

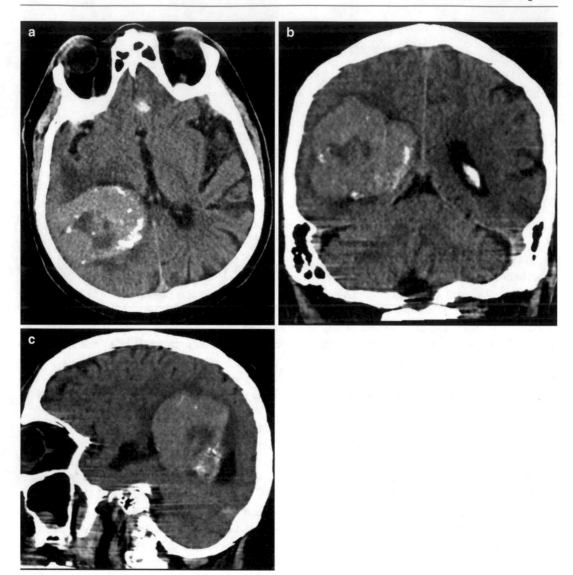

Fig. 16.1 Non-contrast CT exam of the brain. Axial (**a**), coronal (**b**) and sagittal (**c**) reformats. A large, mostly hyperdense, partially calcified mass lesion emerging from the trigone of the right-sided lateral ventricle. Central hypodensity may suggest necrosis. Most likely diagnosis—an intraventricular meningioma

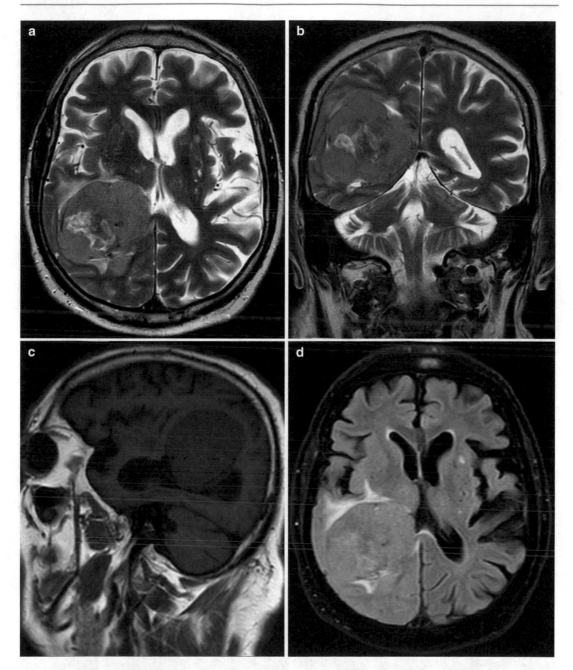

Fig. 16.2 MRI of the brain. Axial (**a**) and coronal (**b**) T2WI, sagittal T1WI (**c**), axial T2-FLAIR (**d**), axial ADC map (**e**) and DWI (**f**), axial post-contrast T1WI (**g**, **h**). A large mass lesion centred at the choroid plexus of the tri-gone of the right-sided lateral ventricle, mostly hypoin-tense in T2WI and well enhanced in post-contrast T1WI, except centrally where signs of hypovascularity are seen. Note mildly decreased diffusion (**e**, **f**) in solid enhanced portions, a feature found in hypercellular tumours such as this meningioma

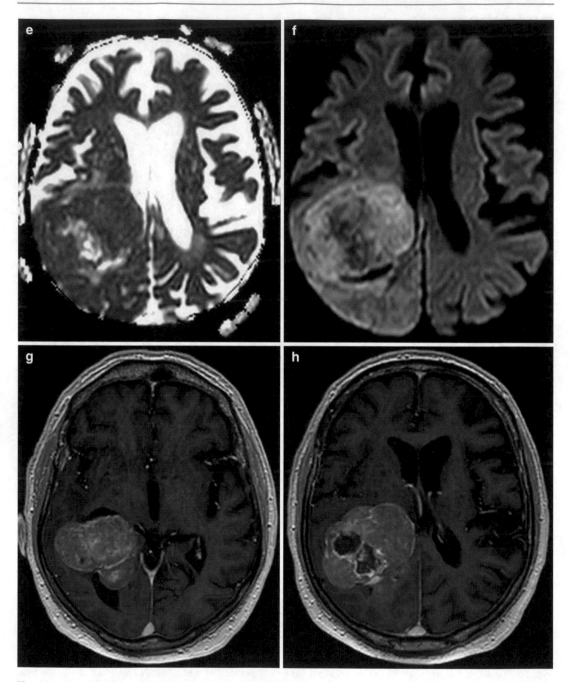

Fig. 16.2 (continued)

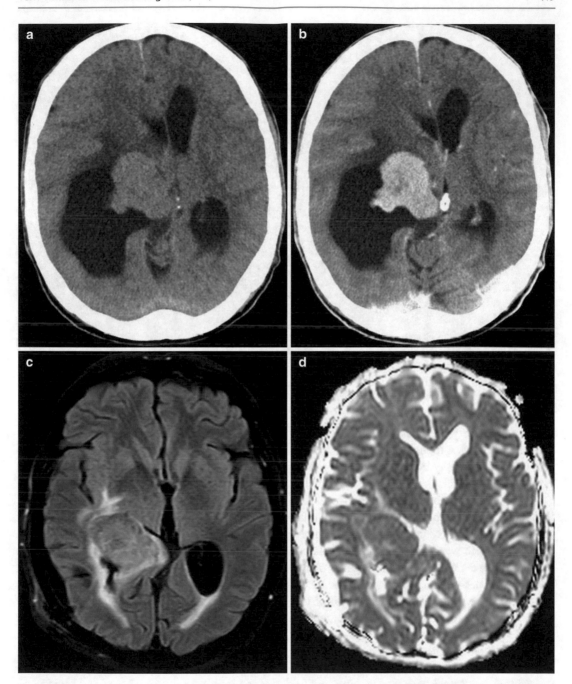

Fig. 16.3 Brain CT (**a**, **b**). Brain MRI (**c**–**f**). Non-contrast (**a**) and contrast-enhanced brain CT. T2-FLAIR (**c**), ADC map (**d**), coronal T2WI (**e**) and axial post-contrast T1WI MR images of the brain. An intraventricular, homogenously enhancing mass lesion in the medial aspect of the right trigone, with marked enlargement of the right-sided trigone and occipital horn. In MR images, the trigone is already decompressed by a shunt (note a linear hypodensity posterolateral to the right ventricular trigone in image **f**). Evidence of vasogenic oedema in the parenchyma adjacent to the tumour. Enhancement, hypointensity in T2WI and mild diffusion impairment suggested a meningioma

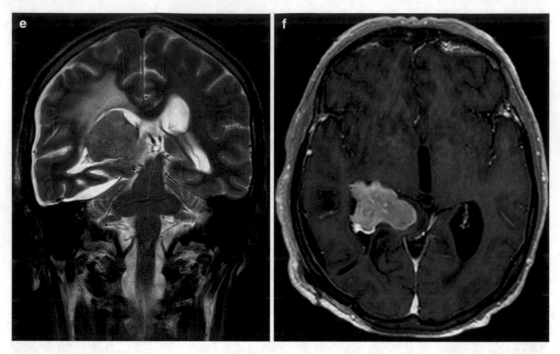

Fig. 16.3 (continued)

motor and sensory, have also been noted [1, 2]. The majority of symptoms are caused by the mass effect causing hydrocephalus or direct compression of the brain.

IVMs arise from the arachnoid cap (outer lining) cells which migrate along with choroid plexus at the time of ventricular system invagination, by the 25th week of gestation. The bulkiest choroid plexuses are sited in the trigones of the lateral ventricles—that is why most of the IVMs are found there. The relatively large size of the trigones allows for significant asymptomatic growth. In terms of histology, IVMs do not differ from other meningiomas. The majority are WHO grade I—meningothelial, fibrous (fibroblastic), transitional or lymphoplasmacyte rich, while only a small number are grade II (atypical) [3]. There have also been sporadic cases of malignant IVMs with distal metastases.

Imaging features of IVMs do not differ from meningiomas in other locations—these are well-defined, highly cellular tumours isodense or hyperdense on CT, isointense to the cerebral grey matter in T1 and T2 weighted images on MR, although some variants demonstrate lower signal intensity in T1- and higher in T2-weighted images. There is vivid contrast enhancement which can be inhomogeneous in cases of tumour infarctions or necrosis. The diffusion is slightly impaired. MR spectroscopy reveals a high choline level and low to non-existent NAA signal, with an alanine doublet (1.3–1.5 ppm). They appear to harbour calcifications more frequently than extraventricular meningiomas. There is often hydrocephalus or a trapped occipital or temporal horn and some vasogenic oedema of the adjacent brain parenchyma. The arterial blood supply of an IVM mainly comes from the posterior choroidal arteries (branches of

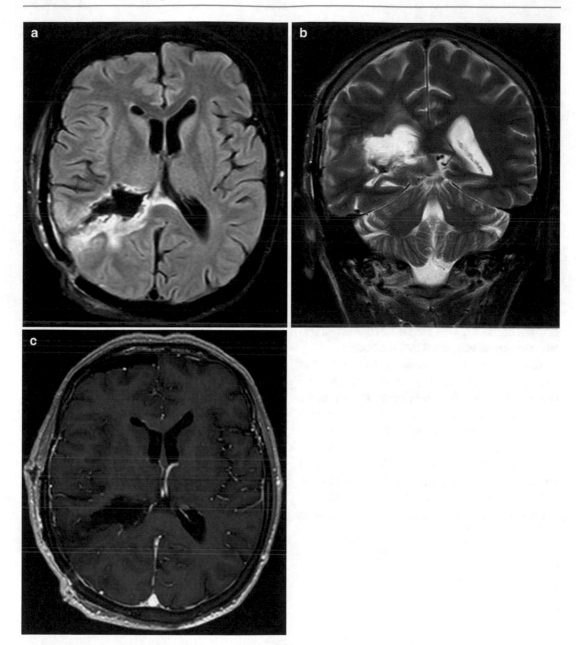

Fig. 16.4 Postoperative MRI of the brain, performed within 48 h after surgery. Axial T2-FLAIR (**a**), coronal T2WI (**b**) and post-contrast axial T1WI (**c**) showing nor- mal post-operative status, without evidence of residual tumour and with regression of vasogenic oedema

the P2 segment of the PCA) and in some cases also from branches of the anterior choroidal artery (originating from the ICA). Catheter angiography is not essential as these tumours are usually not amenable to preoperative embolization [4]—there is a considerable risk of stroke, affecting posterior choroidal arteries territory, causing visual field and sensory loss, although there are case reports of such a procedure [5]. However, catheter angiography may yield information on IVM blood supply and position of the draining veins which is useful during surgery [1]. MR angiography can usually provide information on displacement of the anterior choroidal artery by the tumour. Neuronavigation helps to identify and dissect the supplying vessels during surgery [3].

Differential diagnoses include choroid plexus papilloma, glial tumours (astrocytoma, ependymoma), choroid plexus metastases (renal cell carcinoma, melanoma) and CNS lymphoma.

Gross total resection remains the treatment of choice for the IVMs. Non-adherent margins and benign nature of the IVMs make for a feasible complete microsurgical resection. The challenges are deep location, anatomy of the blood supply and proximity of eloquent brain areas. Superior parietal lobule approach allows for trigonal IVM resection, while temporal horn and inferior trigone may be reached by inferior or middle temporal gyrus approach. Anterior corpus callosum approach is suitable for tumours in frontal horn and body of the lateral ventricle, as well as in the third ventricle, while posterior corpus callosum approach opens a path to a tumour in trigone area. Median suboccipital craniotomy is the preferred route to the fourth ventricle tumour [1].

Tumour recurrence is possible, less likely in low WHO grade tumours. The recurrence of WHO grade II IVMs is most likely in the first 2 years after resection, so MRI evaluation should be performed every 6 months for the first 2 years and annually afterwards.

References

1. Chen C, et al. Clinical features, surgical management, and long-term prognosis of intraventricular meningiomas: a large series of 89 patients at a single institution. Medicine. 2019;98(16):e15334. https://doi.org/10.1097/MD.0000000000015334.
2. Lyngdoh BT, et al. Intraventricular meningiomas: a surgical challenge. J Clin Neurophysiol. 2007;14(5):442–8. https://doi.org/10.1016/j.jocn.2006.01.005.
3. Bertalanffy A, et al. Intraventricular meningiomas: a report of 16 cases. Neurosurg Rev. 2006;29(1):30–5. https://doi.org/10.1007/s10143-005-0414-5.
4. Fusco DJ, Spetzler RF. Surgical considerations for intraventricular meningiomas. World Neurosurg. 2015;83(4):460–1.https://doi.org/10.1016/j.wneu.2014.08.042.
5. Jack AS, et al. Pre-operative embolization of an intraventricular meningioma using onyx. Can J Neurol Sci. 2016;43(1):206–9.

A young man of 32 years of age, previously healthy, was hospitalized in a county hospital on account of multiple motor Jacksonian seizures affecting his left arm, with one secondary generalized seizure. Brain CT reported a mass lesion in the right-sided precentral area (Fig. 17.1).

The patient was transferred to the neurosurgical department of our hospital; on admission, there was mild left-sided weakness. An MRI exam was requested (Fig. 17.2).

The patient underwent surgery for the removal of the mass lesion which was uneventful; there was residual mild left arm and moderate left leg weakness which later improved on physical therapy.

The histopathology findings confirmed the MRI report of a cavernous malformation (cavernoma).

17.1 Cavernoma

Cerebral cavernous venous malformations, known as cavernous haemangiomas or cavernomas, are among the most common cerebral vascular abnormalities, accounting for 10–25% of all cerebral vascular malformations, second only to developmental venous anomalies (DVA) with which they frequently co-exist. The incidence of cavernomas in general population is 0.4–0.8%. Most of them are sited supratentorially (70–80%) [1]. There is no difference in incidence among men and women [2]. Both children and adults may harbour cavernomas.

The International Society for the Study of Vascular Anomalies (ISSVA) classification for vascular anomalies, revision from 2018, classifies cerebral cavernous malformations as slow flow venous malformations in simple vascular malformations III group.

Approximately 40–60% of patients with cavernomas have the familial form, an autosomal dominant heterozygous mutation in one of the three genes, CCM1 (on 7q chromosome, KRIT1 protein abnormality), CCM2 (on 7p chromosome, Malcavernine protein abnormality), and CCM3 (on 3p chromosome, PDCD10 protein abnormality) [1]. In familial form, cavernomas are usually multiple (in 84.6%), while in sporadic form they may be multiple (in 25.4%) [2].

A vast majority of cavernomas are small (15–19 mm) [2]. Giant (>6 cm) cavernomas are very rare [3, 4]. Cavernomas may grow or shrink in time, or even appear de novo [1].

Cavernomas consist of clusters of sinusoidal vascular spaces (caverns) lined only by endothelial cells supported by collagenous matrix, without an elastic lamina or a smooth muscle layer [2, 5]. There is no intervening brain parenchyma. The vessels are irregular in shape and contain blood, thrombi and calcification. Abnormalities in endothelial gap junctions cause recurring microhaemorrhages within the cavernoma. These recurring microhaemorrhages lead to

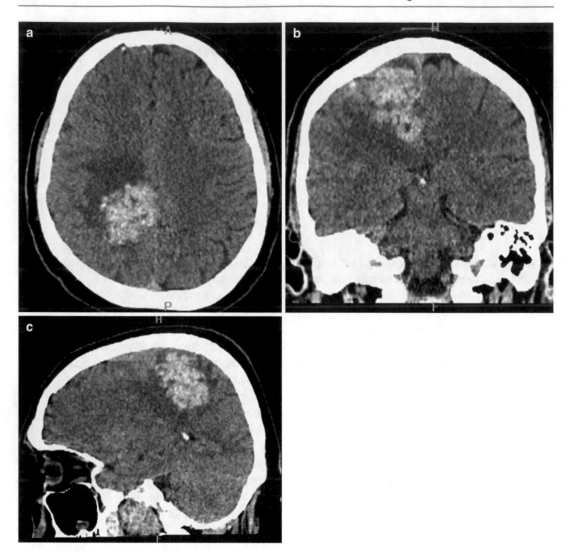

Fig. 17.1 Non-contrast CT exam of the brain—axial (**a**), sagittal (**b**) and coronal (**c**) reformats. A large inhomogenously hyperdense mass lesion in the right-sided precentral area, with some adjacent vasogenic oedema

organization, fibrosis and calcification, may cause slow progressive growth of a cavernoma and are a cause of peripheral haemosiderin deposits and reactive rim of gliosis in the adjacent parenchyma. The blood flow within cavernomas is slow and the pressure is low—that is the reason they are usually not detected angiographically and have a lower risk of rupture compared to some other vascular malformations such as arteriovenous malformations [6].

The annual risk of haemorrhage for supratentorial cavernomas is 0.7–1.1% if there is no history of haemorrhage, but rises to 4.5% in patients with prior intracerebral haemorrhage. The risk of haemorrhage for the infratentorial cavernomas is somewhat higher, reported up to 6.5% per patient-year without prior intraparenchymal haemorrhage and up to 35% (even 60%!) per patient-year with a history of haemorrhage [1]. Also, the risk of haemorrhage is higher in women which may suggest endocrine factors influencing bleeding, especially since oestrogen receptors were detected in a few cavernomas harboured by female patients [2]. Superficial cavernomas carry a lower risk of intracerebral haemorrhage than deeply located cavernomas [1].

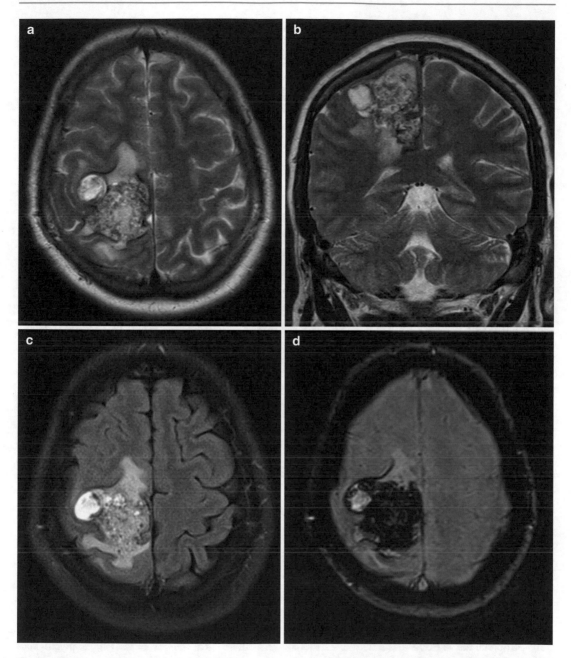

Fig. 17.2 Brain MRI exam—axial (**a**) and coronal (**b**) T2WI, axial T2-FLAIR (**c**), axial SWI sequence (**d–f**) showing an inhomogeneous intra-axial right frontal lobe lesion measuring 42 × 37 × 40 mm, with a haemosiderin rim and internal haemosiderin. MRI spectroscopy revealed no features of tumoral metabolism. Note two small low-intensity lesions on SWI sequence in the left brain hemisphere in (**e**) and (**f**). The findings suggest a haemorrhagic cavernoma in the right frontal lobe

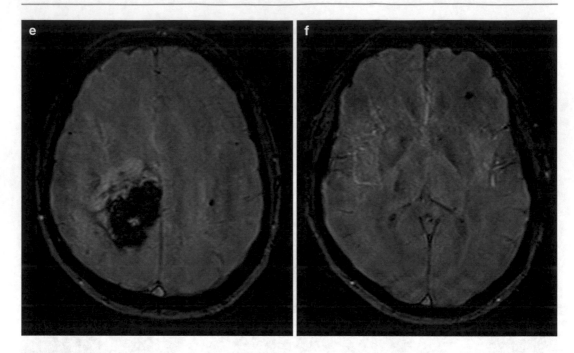

Fig. 17.2 (continued)

Intralesional or perilesional haemorrhage is the usual underlying cause of the neurological deficit; the type of deficit depends on cavernoma/haemorrhage location. There is no distinct pattern of bleeding from a cavernoma—it may range from a microhaemorrhage without clinical and even neuroradiological evidence to a large bleed causing massive neurological deficit and in rare instances even subarachnoid and intraventricular haemorrhage [2]. In non-eloquent brain areas, there may be a clinically silent acute bleed from a cavernoma; on the other hand, brainstem lesions can be symptomatic even without a neuroradiologically visible acute bleed as they may compress nerve tracts and nuclei. Brainstem haemorrhages from cavernomas are symptomatic in 60% of cases, the symptoms usually slowly resolve as the blood is absorbed over time [2]. The most frequent symptoms in patients with brainstem lesions are neuro-ophthalmological, ataxia, hemihypesthesia, cranial nerve (other than oculomotor) deficit, hemiparesis and headache; in most patients symptoms are multiple. Lesions outside the brainstem most commonly present with

seizures, headache and focal neurological deficit, and less than 50% of patients have multiple symptoms [2].

On imaging, the majority of cavernomas are an incidental finding unrelated to patient's symptoms. Therefore, if a well-defined hyperdense round or lobulated lesion, possibly with fine calcifications but without perifocal oedema and mass effect is noted in a non-contrast CT exam of the brain, a diagnosis of cavernoma should be considered. Small cavernomas are difficult to see in CT. In MRI which is the modality of choice, conventional techniques are paramount as flow in cavernomas is not registered by angiographic techniques. Zabramski et al. [7] proposed four types of cavernous malformations based on their MRI appearance: type I lesions contain subacute haemorrhage and appear hyperintense on T1WI, whereas in T2WI they may be either hyper- or hypointense internally but always demonstrate hypointense hemosiderin rim; type II lesions demonstrate mixed signal reflecting various stages of haemorrhage and thrombosis, also with a T2WI hypointense rim; type III lesions contain chronic resolved haemorrhage with haemosiderin within and around the lesion, appear iso- or hypointense in T1WI and hypointense in T2, whereas GRE T2* and SWI sequences demonstrate marked hypointensity with magnification ("blooming") compared to T2WI; type IV are punctate hypointense lesions seen in gradient sequences, while in T1WI and T2WI, they are visualized poorly or not at all. Diffusion tensor imaging provides tractography information which is useful for surgical planning. Functional MRI (fMRI) is also useful preoperatively, but also intraoperatively where available. The use of fMRI neuronavigation provides for a more aggressive surgical approach and yields better results, with more seizure-free patients [1]. Contrast enhancement is often hard to evaluate, generally absent, although possible (Fig. 17.3a, b).

Differential diagnoses, especially for small (type IV) cavernomas, include parenchymal microhaemorrhages seen in chronic hypertensive encephalopathy (periventricular, basal ganglia), cerebral amyloid angiopathy (numerous small foci or amorphous haemosiderin deposits), diffuse axonal injury (DAI), cerebral vasculitis, radiation-induced angiopathy, Parry–Romberg syndrome and haemorrhagic metastases. Larger lesions may be similar to haemorrhagic metastases and primary brain tumours, such as glioblastoma and ependymoma. Calcified infectious lesions such as old cysticercosis should also be considered.

The standard treatment for cavernomas is microsurgical resection. Goals of surgery are to prevent (re)bleeding, to minimize damage to the surrounding tissue and to preserve an associated

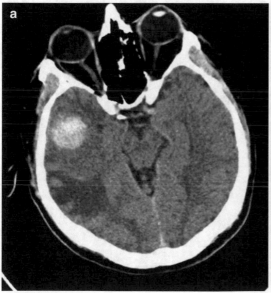
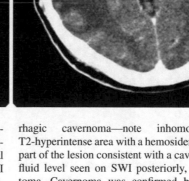

Fig. 17.3 Another patient, admitted to ER with confusion and dysphasia. Non-contrast (**a**) and contrast-enhanced (**b**) brain CT; MRI of the brain (**c–f**)—axial T2WI (**c**) and T2-FLAIR (**d**), axial SWI (**e**), sagittal T1WI (**f**), demonstrating a rather large mass lesion in the right-sided temporal lobe. The CT report stated a haemorrhagic brain tumour. MRI findings consistent with a haemor-rhagic cavernoma—note inhomogeneous, mostly T2-hyperintense area with a hemosiderin rim in the rostral part of the lesion consistent with a cavernoma and a fluid-fluid level seen on SWI posteriorly, within the haematoma. Cavernoma was confirmed both surgically and histopathologically

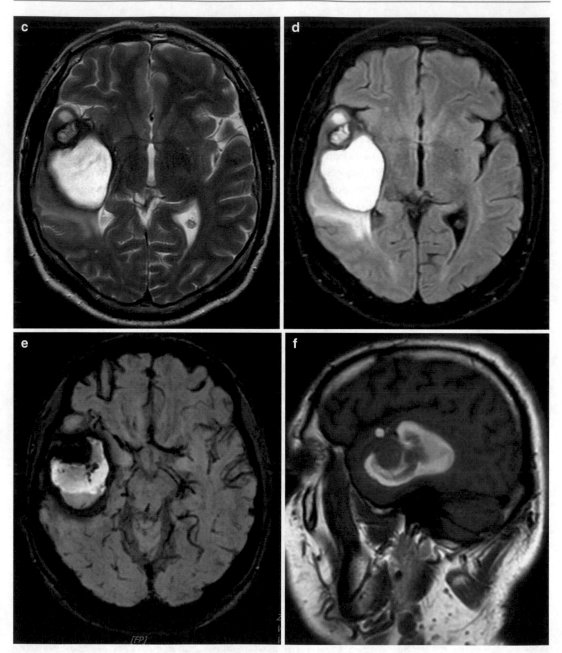

Fig. 17.3 (continued)

DVA if present. However, there is a relatively high risk of complication when resecting cavernomas in deep eloquent locations. The brainstem cavernomas are especially risky to resect. The main criteria for resection of a brainstem cavernoma are severe clinical presentation (haemorrhage included) and location within 2 mm from the pial surface [1]. When the surgical risk is high, stereotactic radiosurgery (SRS) can be used to prevent the natural progression of the lesion. The main goal is significant reduction in bleeding risk, especially after a latency period of 2 years—in that period the SRS exerts it effects, based on the experience with AVMs [2]. Constantly advancing SRS techniques provide less damage to the surrounding tissue while maintaining the desired effect on cavernomas.

Conservative approach consisting of observation and medical treatment where necessary is applied in patients with a known cavernoma who present without specific symptoms, gross haemorrhage or seizures. If a cavernoma is an incidental finding, especially located deeply within functional brain areas, follow-up is also probably the best modality, as well as in cases with multiple lesions. Observation is also applied in patients with non-refractory, medically controlled seizures [2, 5].

References

1. Mouchtouris N, et al. Management of cerebral cavernous malformations: from diagnosis to treatment. TheScientificWorldJOURNAL. 2015;2015:808314. https://doi.org/10.1155/2015/808314.

2. Bertalanffy H, et al. Cerebral cavernomas in the adult. Review of the literature and analysis of 72 surgically treated patients. Neurosurg Rev. 2002;25(1–2):1–53. ; discussion 54–5. https://doi.org/10.1007/s101430100179.

3. van Lindert EJ, et al. Giant cavernous hemangiomas: report of three cases. Neurosurg Rev. 2007;30(1):83–92. ; discussion 92. https://doi.org/10.1007/s10143-006-0042-8.

4. Sharma A, Mittal RS. A giant frontal cavernous malformation with review of literature. J Neurosci Rural Pract. 2016;7(2):279–82. https://doi.org/10.4103/0976-3147.178666.

5. Poeata I, Iencean SM. Cerebral cavernoma. Roman Neurosurg. 2009;16(1):14–7. https://journals.lapub.co.uk/index.php/roneurosurgery/article/view/412.

6. Zyck S, Gould GC. Cavernous venous malformation. [Updated 2020 Feb 21]. In: StatPearls [Internet]. Treasure Island, FL: StatPearls Publishing; 2020. Available from: https://www.ncbi.nlm.nih.gov/books/NBK526009/.

7. Zabramski JM, et al. The natural history of familial cavernous malformations: results of an ongoing study. J Neurosurg. 1994;80(3):422–32. https://doi.org/10.3171/jns.1994.80.3.0422.

Supratentorial Extraventricular Ependymoma vs Arteriovenous Malformation

At the beginning of 2019, a 62-year-old female patient was referred to our hospital for further diagnostic treatment due to symptomatic epilepsy with complex partial seizures. She had a history of arterial hypertension and unregulated diabetes mellitus with diabetic polyneuropathy.

Epileptic seizures lasted periodically for about 2 years, described as paraesthesia and tonic clonic jerks of left extremities followed by a loss of consciousness. Medicamentous treatment of seizures included levetiracetam and lacosamide prescribed by neurologist in another hospital where brain CT was performed in 2017 and 2018. Neither CT images nor radiologist reports were available on patient admission. According to an attending neurologist in our hospital, large, calcified arteriovenous malformation was reported in CT reports. Therefore, neurologist referral for brain MRI was arteriovenous malformation, and I requested for CDs with CT images for comprehensive analysis (Figs. 18.1 and 18.2).

In my opinion, CT revealed supratentorial intra-axial right frontal mass irregular in shape, well-circumscribed, with multiple cysts and extensive calcifications. Content of the cysts was hypodense, but not as CSF, without fluid-fluid levels. Moderate vasogenic oedema surrounded superior part of the mass which compressed frontal horn of the right lateral ventricle, ventral part of the third ventricle and corpus callosum body (Fig. 18.1).

Analysing both CTs, performed in 2017 (Fig. 18.1) and 2018 (Fig. 18.2), I did not find difference in size, shape or other radiomorphological characteristics of the mass. According to available but insufficient medical documentation it was not clear to me on which grounds radiologist based the diagnosis of calcified arteriovenous malformation: MRI, DSA or any kind of intervention have not been performed. As a part of diagnostic work-up during hospitalization in our hospital at the beginning of 2019, MRI of the brain was performed (Figs. 18.3 and 18.4).

After analysing all the aspects of the mass on CT and MRI, I concluded the mass was not a vascular malformation, but primary brain tumour. According to CT (Figs. 18.1 and 18.2) and MRI (Figs. 18.3 and 18.4) radiomorphological appearances and symptom presentation, I concluded that the tumour could be a supratentorial ependymoma clinically presenting with symptomatic epilepsy.

The patient underwent right frontal craniotomy, and the tumour was completely removed: according to intraoperative pathologist consultation, the tumour was ependymoma. After a few days, final pathologist report was ependymoma with numerous calcifications and osseous metaplasia, grade II according to 2016 WHO classification of the CNS tumours.

M. Špero, H. Vavro, *Neuroradiology - Images vs Symptoms*,
https://doi.org/10.1007/978-3-030-69213-1_18

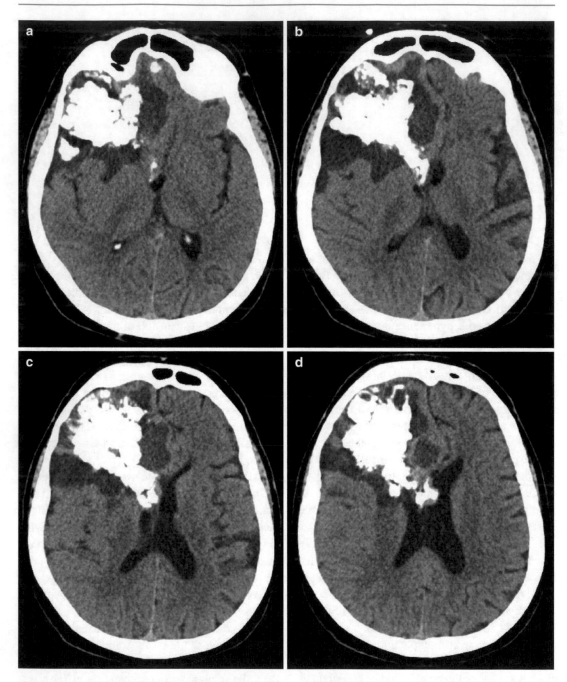

Fig. 18.1 Computed tomography of the brain (non-contrast), performed in another hospital, axial (**a–f**), coronal (**g–l**), sagittal (**m–r**) scans: radiologist reported calcified arteriovenous malformation. Written radiologist report has not been available to me

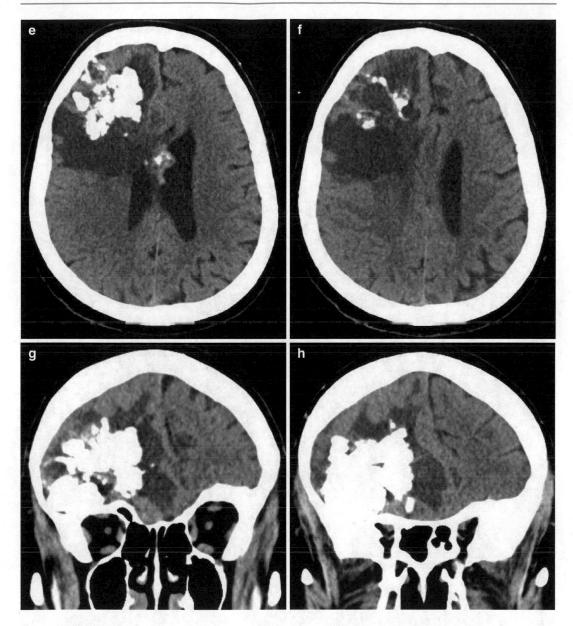

Fig. 18.1 (continued)

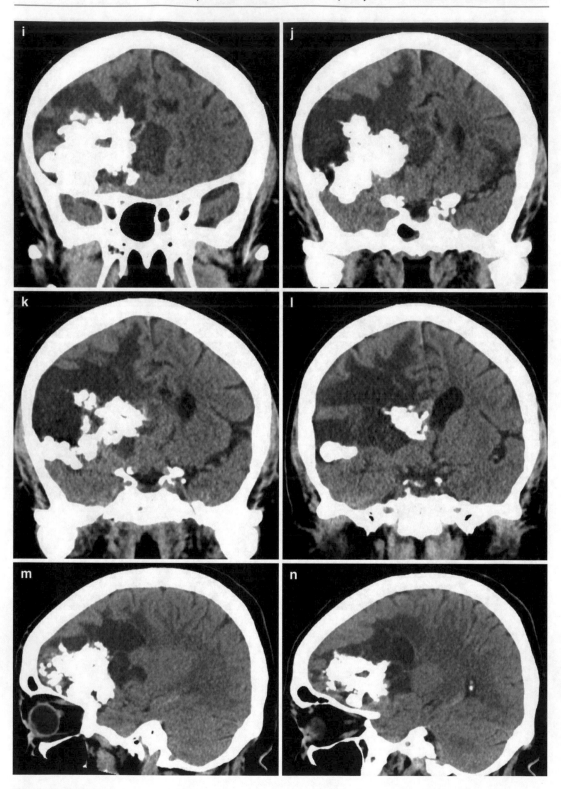

Fig. 18.1 (continued)

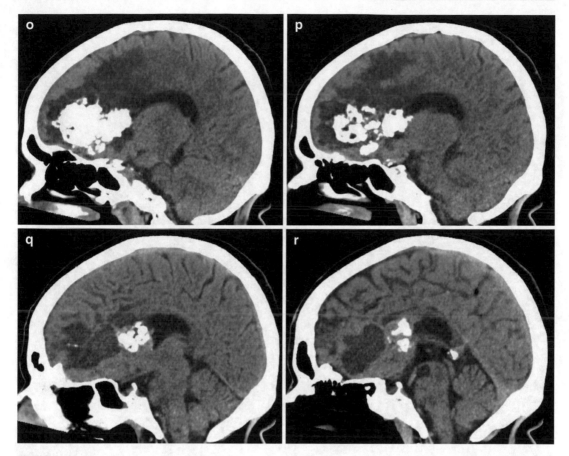

Fig. 18.1 (continued)

18.1 Supratentorial Extraventricular Ependymoma vs Arteriovenous Malformation

Ependymomas are glial tumours derived from differentiated ependymal and subependymal cells lining the ventricles of the brain and the central canal of the spinal cord. They represent approximately 3–9% of all neuroepithelial neoplasms and 6–12% of all paediatric brain tumours [1]. According to the 2016 revision of the WHO classification of CNS tumours, ependymal tumours are divided into Grade I (subependymoma and myxopapillary ependymoma), Grade II (ependymoma) and Grade III (anaplastic ependymoma) [2].

Sixty percent of ependymomas arise infratentorially filling the fourth ventricle, while 40% are supratentorial in location. Supratentorial ependymoma (STE) has no gender predilection, and the peak manifestation is in the adult age group (mean age, 18–24 years) [3].

Supratentorial ependymoma is uncommon, but distinct tumour entity that may be intraventricular or extraventricular intraparenchymal in origin. Supratentorial intraventricular ependymomas may arise from anywhere within the lateral ventricle or third ventricle. Occasionally, they can invade adjacent brain parenchyma and may be associated with CSF metastases to other parts of the ventricular system or to the intracranial or intraspinal subarachnoid space.

Supratentorial extraventricular form arises from the white matter having a predilection for frontal or parietal lobe. The pathogenesis of this type of tumours is uncertain: ependymal cells that extend periventricularly deep into the adja-

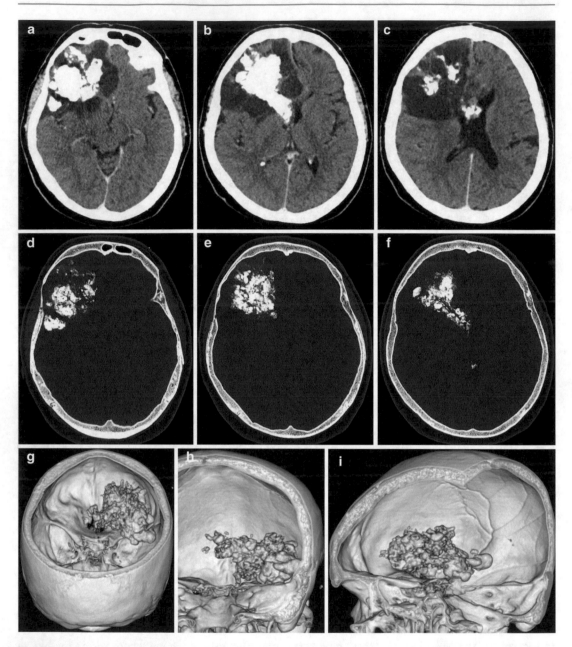

Fig. 18.2 Computed tomography of the brain, post-contrast axial (**a**–**c**) scans, bone window axial (**d**–**f**), volume rendering technique axial (**g**), coronal (**h**), sagittal (**i**), scans: mass did not revealed contrast enhancement. Extensive calcifications ranged from small punctate foci, to serpiginous and massive calcifications. Could calcifications be described as the "periwinkle sign"?

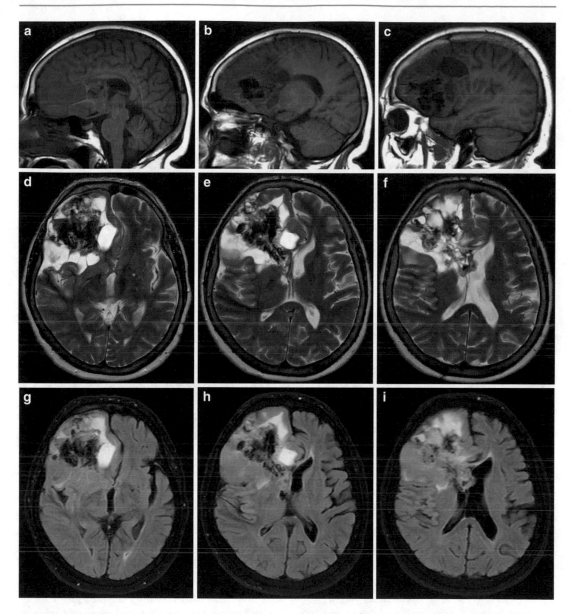

Fig. 18.3 Magnetic resonance imaging of the brain (non-contrast), sagittal T1WI (**a–c**), axial T2WI (**d–f, j**), FLAIR FS (**g–i, m**), SWI (**k, n**), DWI (**l**), ADC (**o**), confirmed supratentorial intra-axial expansile mass involving large part of the right frontal lobe and corpus callosum body. Mass was irregular in shape, well-circumscribed, with moderate perilesional vasogenic oedema surrounding its superior part. The mass itself consisted of large massive confluent calcifications surrounded by cystic part consisting of several cysts different in size and fluid content according to its signal intensity. There were few linear hemosiderin deposits in cysts walls, but no restricted diffusion. The mass compressed frontal horn of the right lateral ventricle and ventral part of the third ventricle

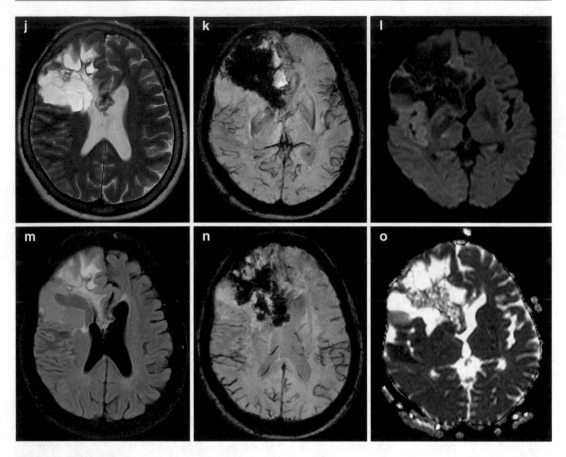

Fig. 18.3 (continued)

cent white matter or foetal remnants of the ependymal cells have been hypothesized to be the cellular origin of these neoplasms. However, the random distribution of ependymomas around the periventricular region in many previous studies makes this hypothesis controversial [4, 5].

There is also a rare, small subset of supratentorial extraventricular ependymomas that selectively involve the cerebral cortex, called cortical ependymomas.

Clinical manifestations of STEs are nonspecific and depend on the tumour location and size. Intraventricular ependymomas usually cause intracranial hypertension, whereas headaches, seizures and local neurosurgical deficits are common in extraventricular STEs [1, 6].

From a radiological point of view, extraventricular STEs are typically large, well-circumscribed masses, possibly spheric in shape: according to

Armington et al. the average size at the time of diagnosis is 4 cm or larger [6]. They are usually cystic masses and may contain calcification ranging from small punctate foci to large masses, especially if low-grade in contrast to high-grade supratentorial ependymoma which is rarely calcified [7].

STEs are iso- to slightly hypoattenuating to surrounding brain parenchyma on non-contrast CT. On MRI, they are iso- to hypointense to normal white matter on unenhanced T1WI and iso- to hyperintense on T2WI. Cystic component could be a simple or complex cyst. Foci of low signal on greT2* or SWI within a neoplasm indicate haemorrhage or calcifications [8].

Term "periwinkle sign" has been designed to describe a characteristic appearance of intraparenchymal supratentorial ependymomas on non-enhanced CT axial images: central solid component with centripetal calcification sur-

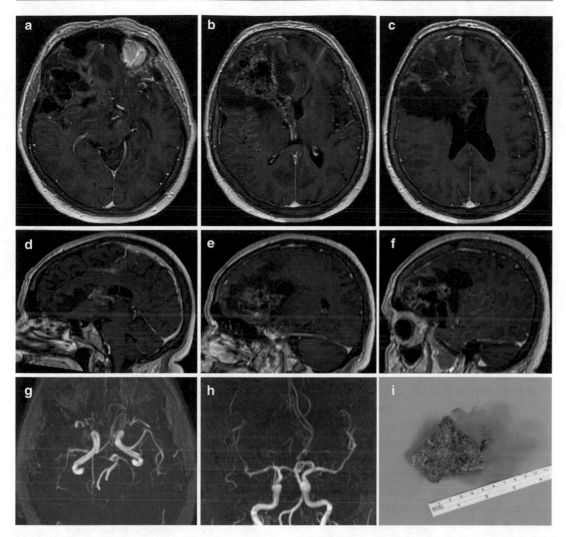

Fig. 18.4 Magnetic resonance imaging of the brain, post-contrast T1WI axial (**a–c**) and sagittal (**d–f**) scans. After intravenous administration of gadolinium contrast media, there was irregular rim contrast enhancement in the central part of the mass which was hypointense on all non-contrast sequences—"bubbly like" pattern of the contrast enhancement. There were no contrast enhancement in the walls of cysts. There was discreet cortical contrast enhancement involving right inferior frontal gyrus behind the mass and superior frontal gyrus above the mass, revealing restricted diffusion indicating possible subacute ischaemia due to parenchymal hypoperfusion. Magnetic resonance angiography (3D TOF technique) (**g, h**) did not reveal arteriovenous malformation. Gross pathology of the removed mass (**i**) (courtesy of D. Romić, specialist in neurosurgery): for the most part, the mass was calcified

rounding central necrotic area resembles a flower. Often present surrounding peripheral cyst is imagined to be a leaf [3].

Heterogeneous moderate to intense enhancement of the solid component and enhancement of cyst margins are noted on CT and MRI. Cystic with mural nodule pattern of contrast enhancement on MRI could be present in hemispheric location of such tumours [9, 10]. Associated secondary finding includes peritumoural oedema.

On advanced imaging such as diffusion sequence, areas of hypercellular solid portions reveal restricted diffusion. MRS with short TE described in a series revealed increased glutamine and glutamate. Perfusion MRI using T2*-weighted dynamic susceptibility has been described in STE and demonstrated markedly elevated CBV with a poor return to baseline. The rCBV was increased approximately five times more in our case with Grade III tumour. This has been attributable to fenestrated blood vessels and an incomplete blood–brain barrier [8].

The differential diagnosis of supratentorial extraventricular ependymomas includes pilocytic astrocytoma, glioblastoma multiforme, ganglioglioma, pleomorphic xanthoastrocytoma, and oligodendroglioma.

The 5- and 10-year survival rates for adults with supratentorial ependymomas are 57.1% and 45%, respectively [11].

Gross total or maximal safe resection with adjuvant radiotherapy is the current mainstay of treatment [10–12]. A postoperative MRI with contrast is recommended for further evaluation of the extent of resection. It is worth mentioning that some authors recommend adjuvant radiotherapy if the tumour is cystic, even after apparently total resection [11].

It was not easy for me to make a correct diagnose in this particular case. Although neurologist referral for the brain MRI was arteriovenous malformation, I could not find any evidence for such vascular malformation on MRI (Figs. 18.3 and 18.4a–f) and MRA (Fig. 18.4g, h), as well as on prior head CTs (Figs. 18.1 and 18.2). I reported large supratentorial extraventricular mass involving large part of the right frontal lobe that consisted of central large masses of calcification surrounded with several cysts and moderate perilesional oedema showing moderate inhomogeneous "bubbly"-like appearance of contrast enhancement. It could only be a primary tumour: after summing clinical presentation and all radio-morphological characteristics, I conclude it could be a supratentorial extraventricular ependymoma. Neither one of the other previously mentioned differential diagnoses did not fit due to radiological appearance of the process as well as symptom presentation. Whether large masses of calcifica-

tion fit the "periwinkle sign" on non-contrast axial CT images I am not sure. The patient underwent right frontal craniotomy, and the tumour was completely removed. The surgery itself went well without complications, but postoperative course was complicated by haemorrhage filling postoperative cavity: it was drained twice, but unfortunately, at the end, the patient did not survive.

References

1. Mermuys K, et al. Best cases from the AFIP supratentorial ependymoma. Radiographics. 2005;25(2):486–90.
2. Louis DN, et al. The 2016 World Health Organization classification of tumors of the central nervous system: a summary. Acta Neuropathol. 2016;131:803–20.
3. Mangalore S, et al. Imaging characteristics of supratentorial ependymomas: study on a large single institutional cohort with histopathological correlation. Asian J Neurosurg. 2015;10(4):276–81.
4. Sun S, et al. Clinical, radiological, and histological features and treatment outcomes of supratentorial extraventricular ependymoma: 14 cases from a single center. J Neurosurg. 2018;128(5):1396–402.
5. Wang M, et al. Supratentorial cortical ependymomas: a retrospective series of 13 cases at a single center. World Neurosurg. 2018;112:772–7.
6. Armington WG, et al. Supratentorial ependymoma: CT appearance. Radiology. 1985;157:367–72.
7. Lefton DR, et al. MRI features of intracranial and spinal eypendimomas. Pediatr Neurosurg. 1998;28:97–105.
8. Yuh EL, et al. Imaging of ependymomas: MRI and CT. Chikls Nerv Syst. 2009;25:1203–13.
9. Shuangshoti S, et al. Supratentorial extraventricular ependymal neoplasms a clinicopathologic study of 32 patients. Cancer. 2005;103(12):2598–605.
10. Ng DWK, et al. Anaplastic supratentorial cortical ependymoma presenting as a butterfly lesion. Surg Neurol Int. 2012;3:107.
11. Rebai R, et al. Intra parenchymal extraventricular supratentorial ependymomas: case report and review of pathophysiology and management. J Med Cases. 2013;4(4):237–41.
12. Han MH, et al. Supratentorial extraventricular anaplastic ependymoma presenting with repeated intratumoral hemorrhage. Brain Tumor Res Treat. 2014;2(2):81–6.

Pachymeningial Involvement in Acute Myeloid Leukaemia (AML)

A 53-year-old male was urgently hospitalized in our facility because of seizures and severe thrombocytopenia. If you have read Chap. 14 of this very book, you might already have an idea about what it was, but no—this was not another case of TTP because, well, we already have a chapter on that. He had been diagnosed with a myelodysplastic syndrome (MDS-RAEB2) which a year later transitioned into acute myeloid leukaemia (AML). His comorbidities included chronic hepatitis B infection, type 2 diabetes, arterial hypertension and an aggressive form of prostatic adenocarcinoma with bone metastases. It was concluded that he was not a candidate for a high-dose chemotherapy nor for an allogeneic stem cell transplantation. He was started on cytoreductive therapy with hydroxyurea, with later addition of thioguanine, supported by platelet and RBC concentrate transfusions twice a week.

On admission his WBC was 20.8×10^9, RBC 2.89×10^{12}, platelet count 41×10^9, haemoglobin 85 g/L—findings consistent with leukocytosis with anaemia and thrombocytopenia.

The patient was referred to head CT (Fig. 19.1) which demonstrated a subdural haematoma—or something else? A contrast-enhanced head CT was beneficial (Fig. 19.2).

The patient deteriorated, with focal motor seizures and cognitive disturbance, head and eyes deviated to the left. Surgical therapy was dismissed by a neurosurgeon. Eight doses of platelet concentrate were applied. The next day, there

was onset of fever. Symptomatic and systemic therapy did not stop the rapid general deterioration of the patient's health, and he unfortunately passed away 36 hours after being admitted to the hospital.

19.1 Central Nervous System (CNS) Involvement in Acute Myeloid Leukaemia (AML)

Acute myeloid leukaemia (AML) originates from precursor tumour-transformed hematopoietic cells, with accumulation of clonal, proliferative, abnormally and occasionally poorly differentiated cells of the hematopoietic system [1]. It used to have a dismal prognosis, but nowadays poor outcome with median survival of only 5–10 months is inevitable only in elderly patients who cannot withstand intensive chemotherapy and its side effects. AML can be cured in 35–40% of adult patients younger than 60 years of age and in 5–15% of patients older than 60 years. In adult patients, AML rarely involves CNS, in contrast to acute lymphoblastic leukaemia (ALL), but it is somewhat more common in paediatric patients. The estimated percentage of CNS involvement in AML is around 5% [2]. At initial diagnosis of AML, CNS infiltration is found in 0.6% of adult patients [3]. CNS involvement may consist of leukaemic blasts in the CSF, cranial nerve involvement with signs of paralysis, myeloid

M. Špero, H. Vavro, *Neuroradiology - Images vs Symptoms*,
https://doi.org/10.1007/978-3-030-69213-1_19

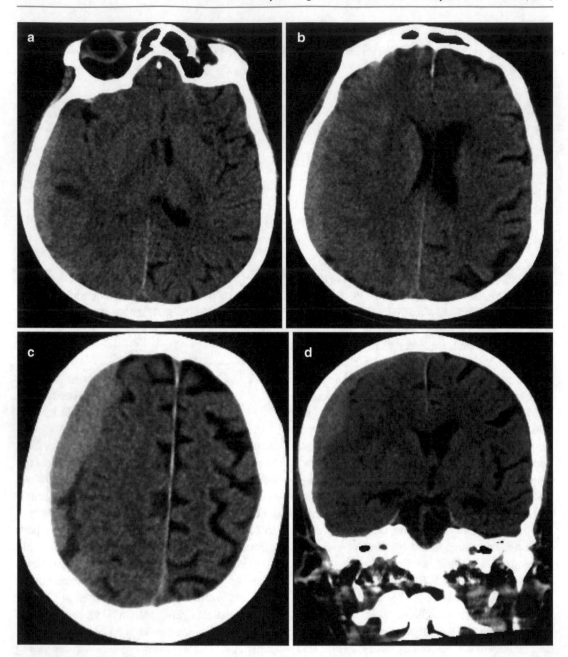

Fig. 19.1 Non-contrast head CT: an extra-axial hyperdense lesion on the right, with mass effect. In a patient with severe thrombocytopenia? This is probably a subdural haematoma. Wait…is it really? The patient is anaemic, his haemoglobin concentration is low—a haematoma in this setting would not be as hyperdense. Let us apply intravenous contrast and see what happens (Fig. 19.2)

sarcoma infiltration of the meninges, brain and/or spinal cord and meningeal AML [3, 4]. The identified risk factors are initially high WBC count in the peripheral blood, higher lactate dehydroge- nase (LDH) levels, complex karyotype and AML M4 or M5 (acute myelomonocytic or monocytic leukaemia) French–American–British (FAB) morphology [3]. Additional risk factors for CNS

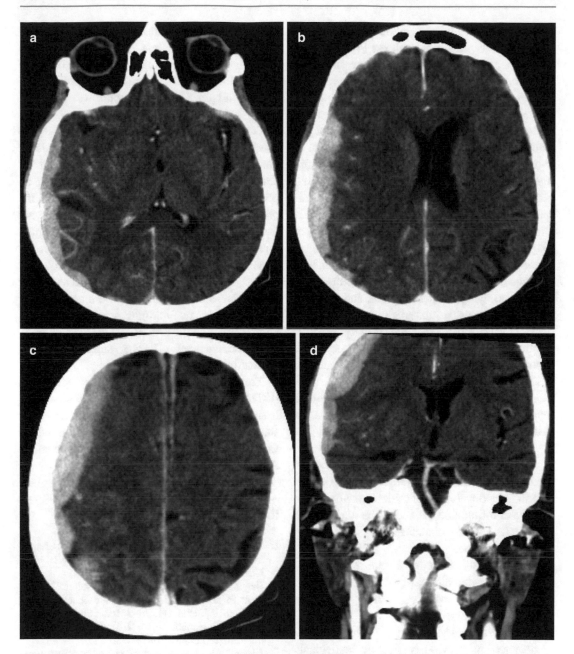

Fig. 19.2 Contrast-enhanced head CT (**a–d**): vivid enhancement of the extra-axial mass on the right. This is definitely not a haematoma, but it definitely could be a dural myeloid sarcoma (see text)

involvement include relapse of the disease and prior CNS or extramedullary infiltration. Cheng et al. in a large retrospective study [5] concluded that the risk factors significantly associated with CNS involvement included age ≤45 years, WBC counts ≥50 × 10^9/L, and the presence of 11q23 chromosomal abnormalities. There seems to be

no gender nor age predilection compared to AML patients without CNS involvement [2].

Symptoms of CNS involvement in AML are varied, many patients are asymptomatic, with only CSF positive for leukaemic blasts. Relapse patients are more prone to intracerebral and cranial nerve involvement and associated symptoms, e.g. cranial nerve palsies, motor deficits, pares-thesiae and asymmetrical reflexes [4]. The most common presentation symptoms are headache and altered mental state - non-specific symptoms caused by increased intracranial pressure or space-occupying effects of myeloid sarcoma.

Myeloid sarcoma (chloroma, granulocytic sarcoma or extramedullary myeloid tumour) is composed of myeloid precursor cells (immature myeloblasts) and may precede bone marrow and peripheral blood disease which makes the accurate diagnosis difficult as its CT and MRI appearance has a broad differential diagnosis. Proper diagnosis of myeloid sarcoma can only be made in correlation with clinical history and laboratory findings [6]. It most frequently affects the bone, periosteum, lymph nodes and skin, and there are reports of less usual presentations in the breast, ovary, rectum, pancreas and urinary bladder. Myeloid sarcoma of the CNS is very rare, accounting for 3.25% of all myeloid sarcoma cases [7].

Audouin et al. [8] proposed classification of myeloid sarcomas (MS) into four varied patterns:

1. Concurrent with AML in the active phase of the disease (the most common pattern).
2. MS that develops alongside known chronic myeloproliferative disorders, the tumour may be the first manifestation of blastic transformation.
3. MS as manifestation of a relapse months or years following clinical remission from AML, particularly after bone marrow transplantation.
4. MS preceding AML diagnosis, which may be detected in previously healthy individuals with no other signs of leukaemia; AML may occur weeks, months or years later. This pattern is often missed.

Immunohistochemistry is essential in diagnosing myeloid sarcoma. CD68-KP1 is the most commonly expressed marker. MPO is a marker expressed in majority of MSs, only some minimally differentiated and monocytic tumours do not express it. Immunohistochemical detection of intracellular MPO confirms the diagnosis. Other common markers include CD117, CD99, CD68/PG M1, lysozyme, CD34, TdT, CD56, CD61/linker of activated T lymphocyte/factor VIII-related antigen, CD30, glycophorin A and CD4 [9].

On imaging, myeloid sarcoma of the CNS is usually a hyperdense, less frequently isodense dural and subperiosteal mass on non-contrast CT scan, vividly and homogenously enhancing on postcontrast scans. If there is disruption of the pial-glial barrier, it infiltrates the underlying brain parenchyma. Bone destruction is not a feature of CNS-MS. MRI appearance is typically hypointense to isointense on T1- and T2-weighted images, with marked post-contrast enhancement [6, 7]. These features are also common in other lesions, such as meningioma, schwannoma, lymphoma (including primary dural lymphoma), while unenhanced CT may suggest subdural haematoma.

Treatments such as high-dose cytarabine (HiDAC), intrathecal chemotherapy and cranial irradiation are effective, but remission times are short and relapse rate is high which along with a short survival time makes CNS involvement in AML a poor prognostic factor [2, 4].

References

1. Döhner H, et al. Acute myeloid leukemia. N Engl J Med. 2015;373(12):1136–52. https://doi.org/10.1056/NEJMra1406184.
2. Bar M, et al. Central nervous system involvement in acute myeloid leukemia patients undergoing hematopoietic cell transplantation. Biol Blood Marrow Transplant. 2015;21(3):546–51. https://doi.org/10.1016/j.bbmt.2014.11.683.
3. Alakel N, et al. Symptomatic central nervous system involvement in adult patients with acute myeloid leukemia. Cancer Manag Res. 2017;9:97–102. https://doi.org/10.2147/CMAR.S125259.
4. Patkowska E, et al. Primary and secondary central nervous system involvement in acute myeloid leukemia. J Leuke. 2019;7:257. https://doi.org/10.24105/2329-6917.7.257.
5. Cheng C-L, et al. Risk factors and clinical outcomes of acute myeloid leukaemia with central nervous system involvement in adults. BMC Cancer. 2015;15:344. https://doi.org/10.1186/s12885-015-1376-9.

6. Cervantes GM, Cayci Z. Intracranial CNS manifestations of myeloid sarcoma in patients with acute myeloid leukemia: review of the literature and three case reports from the author's institution. J Clin Med. 2015;4(5):1102–12. https://doi.org/10.3390/jcm4051102.

7. Yang B, et al. Clinicoradiological characteristics, management and prognosis of primary myeloid sarcoma of the central nervous system: a report of four cases. Oncol Lett. 2017;14(3):3825–31. https://doi.org/10.3892/ol.2017.6620.

8. Audouin J, et al. Myeloid sarcoma: clinical and morphologic criteria useful for diagnosis. Int J Surg Pathol. 2003;11(4):271–82. https://doi.org/10.1177/106689690301100404.

9. Singh A, et al. Unravelling chloroma: review of imaging findings. Br J Radiol. 2017;90(1075):20160710. https://doi.org/10.1259/bjr.20160710.

Part III

Sensory and Motor Deficit

At the end of January 2018, a 68-year-old male patient presented with right hand weakness that lasted for 2 days.

Two years ago, the patient had an episode of a transient ischaemic attack manifested with tingling of the right half of face and right hand and transient right hand weakness. Symptoms lasted for about an hour, resolved completely and did not recur after the episode. The patient was hospitalized, brain CT was performed twice and did not reveal morphological changes like acute ischaemia, haemorrhage or brain tumour. The patient had a history of arterial hypertension.

In 2018, brain CT was performed on admission and reported by general radiologist who was on call. Lesion in the left precentral gyrus was reported as an acute ischaemia (Fig. 20.1). A day later, post-contrast CT of the brain was performed, neuroradiologist analysed it, reported expansile intra-axial lesion matching brain tumour in the left precentral gyrus and recommended MRI of the brain.

After analysis of the brain MRI, neuroradiologist reported primary brain tumour probably high-grade glioma—glioblastoma, or solitary metastasis (Figs. 20.2 and 20.3).

The patient underwent left parietal craniotomy, and the tumour was completely removed: final pathologist report was gliosarcoma, grade IV according to 2016 WHO classification of the CNS tumours. Afterwards chemotherapy and irradiation treatment were conducted. Antiepileptic therapy was introduced due to focal motoric seizures in the right hand after neurosurgical procedure.

Fifteen months after the operation, follow-up MRI did not revealed recurrent tumour: radiation-induced leukoencephalopathy was reported in the white matter of left the parietal and frontal lobes surrounding small postoperative malacia with adjacent gliosis (Fig. 20.4).

Three months after the patient started to show behaviour changes, he was often confused and had intermittent weakness in the legs. MRI of the brain was performed and revealed new, large tumour in the anterior and medial part of the left frontal lobe, involving the body of the corpus callosum. MRI findings (Fig. 20.5) were consistent with high-grade glioma, glioblastoma or secondary gliosarcoma. Postoperative changes in the left postcentral gyrus did not revealed difference in size, shape or signal intensities, as well as no contrast enhancement that could point to gliosarcoma recurrence. The patient underwent left frontal craniotomy and subtotal tumour reduction: final pathologist report was glioblastoma, grade IV according to 2016 WHO classification of the CNS tumours. Prognosis was poor, and the patient died after few months.

M. Špero, H. Vavro, *Neuroradiology - Images vs Symptoms*,
https://doi.org/10.1007/978-3-030-69213-1_20

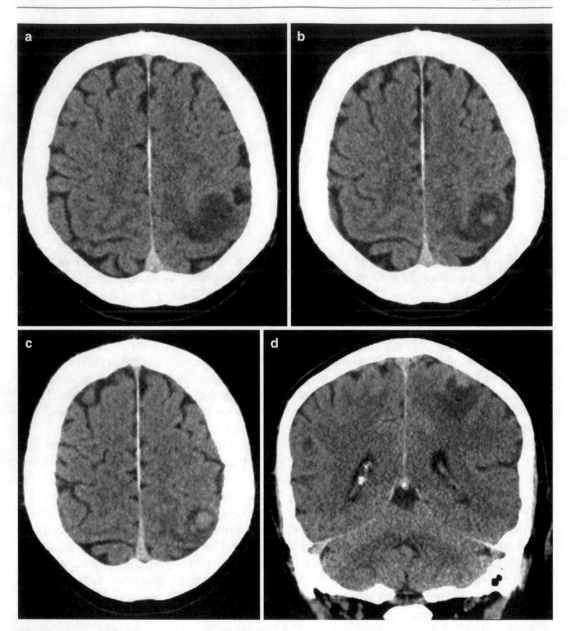

Fig. 20.1 Computed tomography of the brain, performed on admission, non-contrast, axial (**a–c**), coronal (**d–f**), sagittal (**g–i**) scans, revealed hypodense lesion in the left precentral gyrus with narrow surrounding sulci which was reported as an acute ischemia. Small, round, slightly hyperdense part of the lesion was not described in the report made by radiologist on call. Post-contrast CT of the brain (**j–l**), performed a day later, revealed round homogeneous contrast enhancement within the hypodense lesion in the precentral gyrus and very discreet ring-like, contrast enhancement surrounding hypodense part, suggesting brain tumour

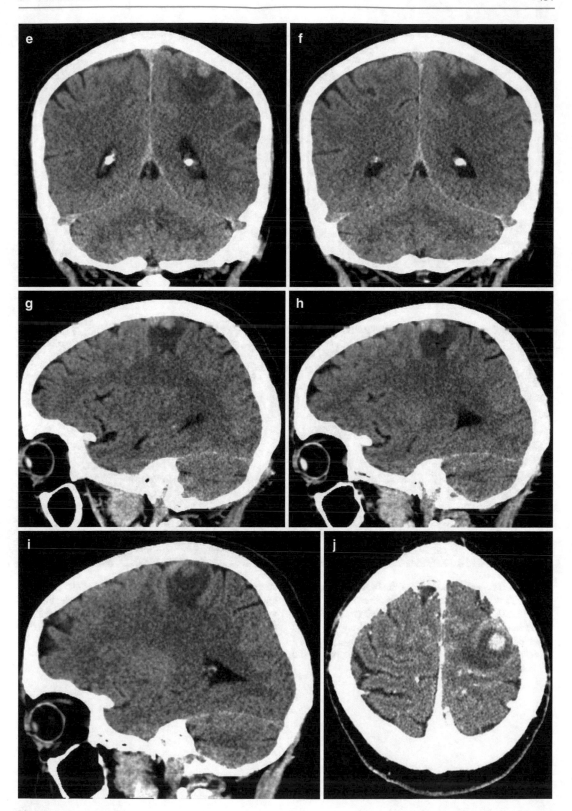

Fig. 20.1 (continued)

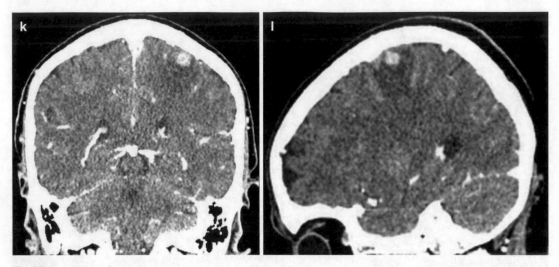

Fig. 20.1 (continued)

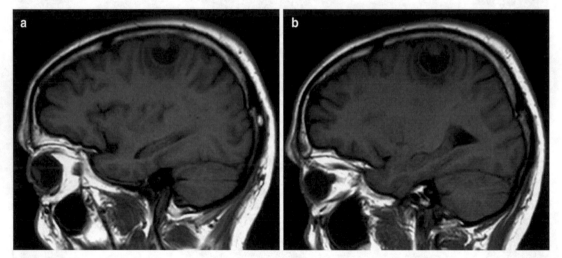

Fig. 20.2 Magnetic resonance of the brain, non-contrast, sagittal T1WI (**a–c**), axial (**d, e**) and coronal (**f, i**) T2WI, axial FLAIR FS (**g, h**), DWI (**j, k**), ADC (**m, n**), SWI (**l, o**), revealed supratentorial, left frontal, well-circumscribed mass peripherally located in the precentral gyrus, surrounded with mild vasogenic oedema. Mass had cystic component with intraluminal mural nodule along the upper part of the cyst wall that abutted dura. Regular cyst wall and intramural nodule showed slightly restricted diffusion. A few punctate hypointensities in the mural nodule on SWI were probably due to microhaemorrhage

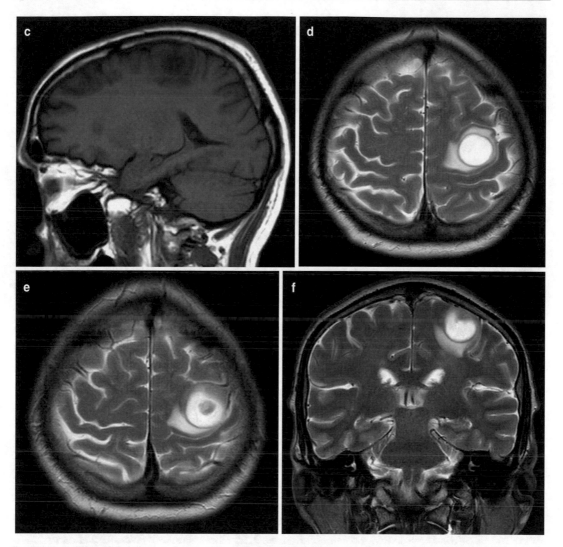

Fig. 20.2 (continued)

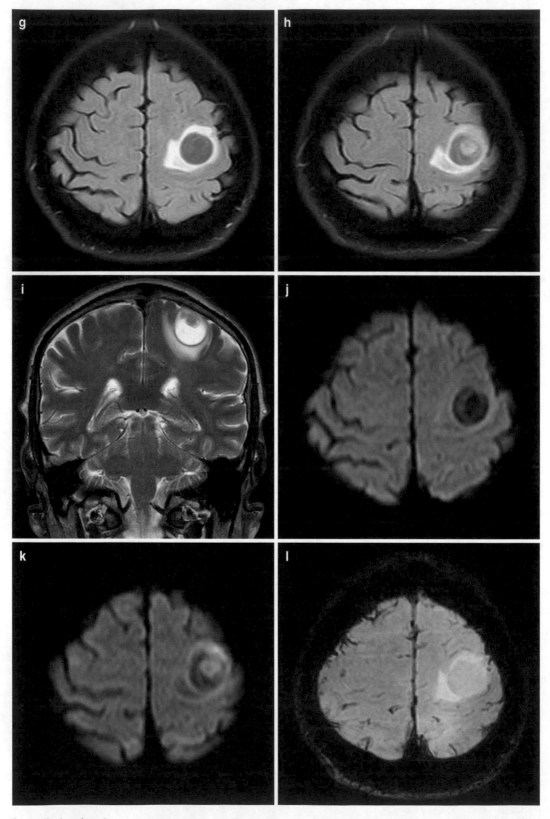

Fig. 20.2 (continued)

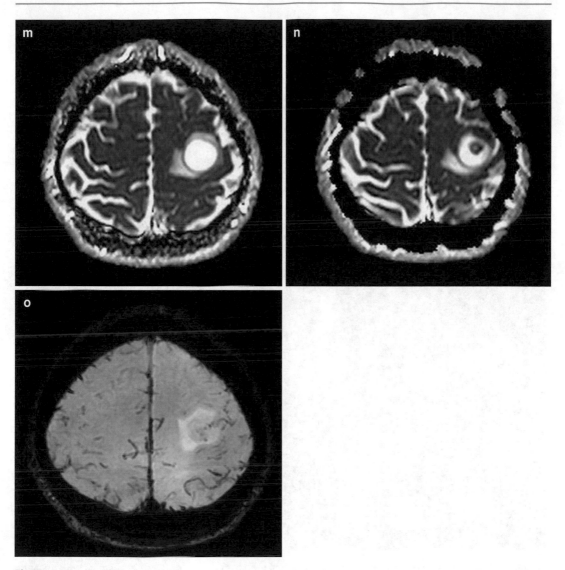

Fig. 20.2 (continued)

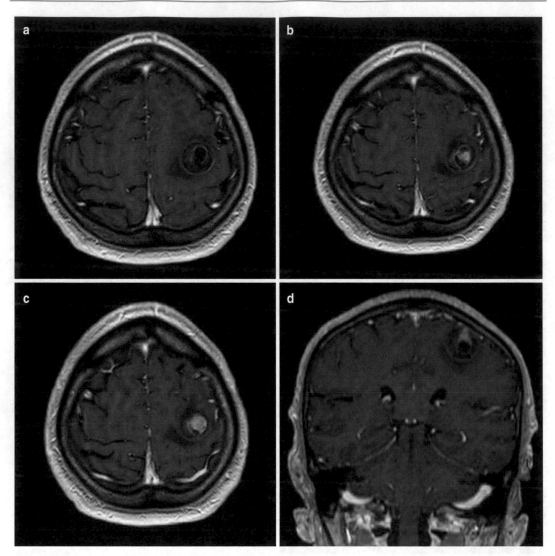

Fig. 20.3 Magnetic resonance imaging of the brain, post-contrast T1WI MPRAGE, axial (**a–c**), coronal (**d–f**), sagittal (**g–i**): expansile mass demonstrated mural nodule with smaller cyst and larger cyst surrounding it. Walls of the both cysts demonstrated regular, ring-like contrast enhancement. Mural nodule demonstrated slightly inhomogeneous contrast enhancement and abutted adjacent dura

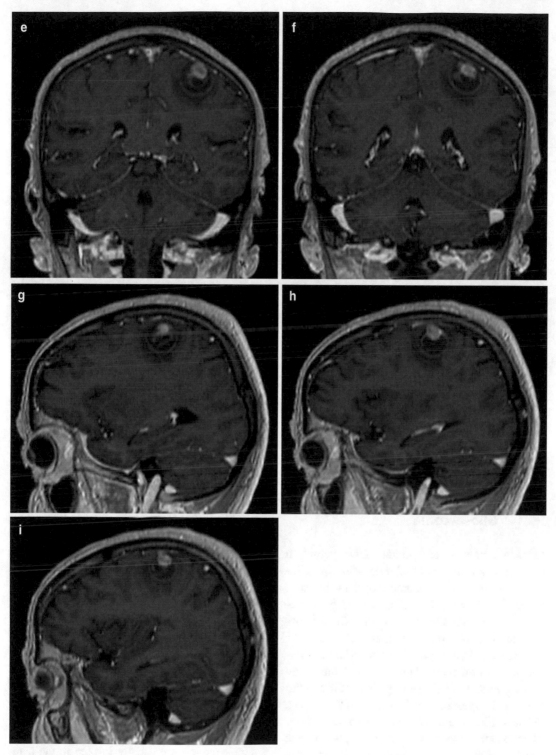

Fig. 20.3 (continued)

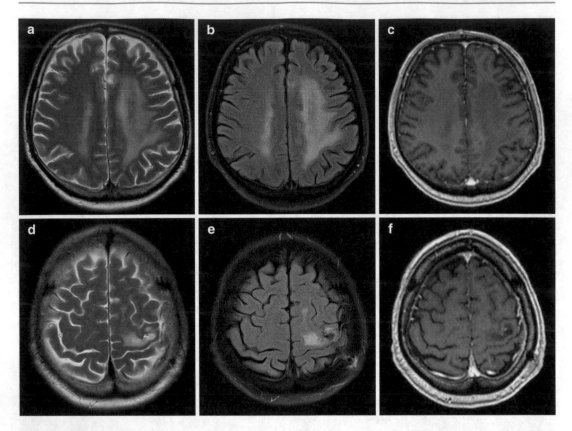

Fig. 20.4 Follow-up magnetic resonance imaging of the brain performed 15 months after craniotomy: axial T2WI (**a**, **d**) and FLAIR FS (**b**, **e**) and post-contrast axial T1WI MPRAGE (**c**, **f**), revealed small postoperative malacia with adjacent gliosis in the precentral gyrus (**a**, **b**, **d**, **e**) without contrast enhancement indicating recurrent tumour (**c**, **f**). Radiation-induced leukoencephalopathy in the surrounding left frontal and parietal white matter (**a–c**)

20.1   Gliosarcoma

Gliosarcoma is a rare primary CNS neoplasm defined as a rare variant of IDH wild-type glioblastoma multiforme characterized by biphasic tissue patterns with alternating areas of both gliomatous and sarcomatous elements. The gliomatous component consists of anaplastic astrocytic tumour cells like in glioblastoma, while the sarcomatous component shows signs of malignant transformation of cells with epithelial differentiation and mesenchymal differentiation [1]. Primary gliosarcoma arise de novo without prior glioblastoma, whereas secondary gliosarcoma occurs after the treatment of conventional glioblastoma.

Incidence of gliosarcoma is of 1–8% of all the malignant gliomas, affecting adult population in the fourth to the sixth decade of life with slight male predominance [2]. It was first reported in 1895 by Heinrich Strobe, a pathologist who worked at Freiburg University Hospital [3], but did not gain wide acceptance until 1955 when Feigen and Gross described it in three patients. They defined gliosarcomas as GBM in which the proliferating vessels had acquired the features of a sarcoma [4]. This "collision tumour" concept is not supported by recent studies which point to a monoclonal origin of both components of gliosarcoma, with sarcomatous component originating through aberrant mesenchymal differentiation of the malignant glioma [5].

Gliosarcomas are usually located in the cerebral cortex demonstrating slight predilection for temporal lobe, but involve frontal, parietal, and occipital lobes as well [6, 7]. Clinical presentation

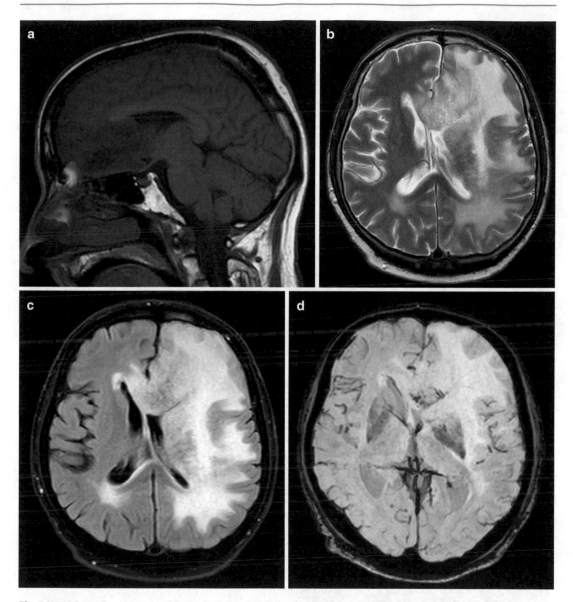

Fig. 20.5 Magnetic resonance of the brain 3 months after the previous follow-up MRI, sagittal T1WI (**a**), axial T2WI (**b**) and FLAIR FS (**c**), SWI (**d**), DWI (**e**), ADC (**f**), and post-contrast sagittal (**g**), axial (**h**) and coronal (**i**) T1WI. Large tumour in the anterior and medial part of the left frontal lobe, involving the body of the corpus callosum was hypointense on T1WI, showed heterogeneous signal intensities on T2WI and FLAIR FS, mild micro-haemorrhage on SWI, slightly restricted diffusion in the solid parts of the mass and inhomogeneous peripheral contrast enhancement with central necrosis on post-contrast T1WI. Extensive vasogenic oedema surrounded tumour that revealed increased rCBV on MR perfusion, and increased cholin and creatine levels, decreased NAA on MR spectroscopy

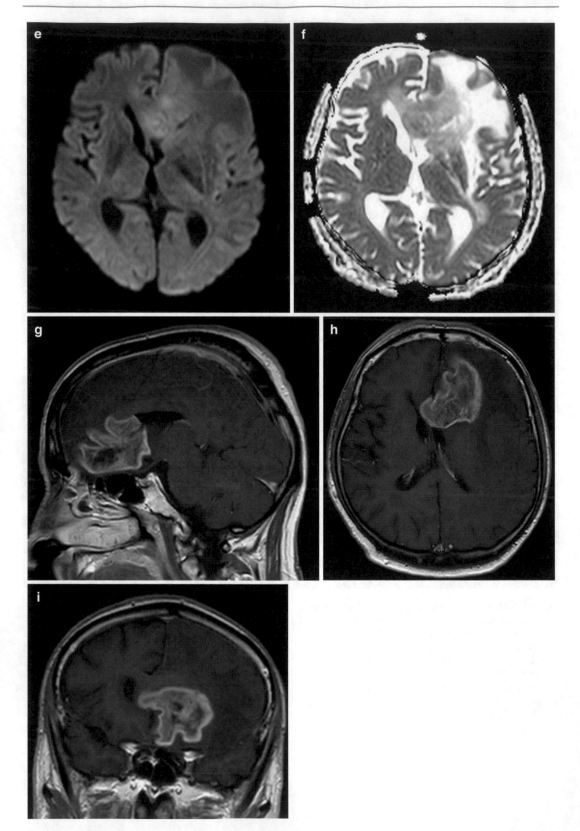

Fig. 20.5 (continued)

depends upon tumour location, while invariably clinical history of the patient is short. It usually includes changes in the level of consciousness, nausea, vomiting and headache, reflecting the compressive aspect resulting from the rapid growth of the tumour surrounded by vasogenic oedema.

Based on clinical or radiological findings we cannot accurately distinguish between gliosarcoma and glioblastoma: diagnostic confirmation is achieved with a histopathological examination.

According to the literature, gliosarcomas are usually described as supratentorial intracranial tumours, peripherally located and often abutting dura. Such tumours are well-defined, surrounded by mild-to-moderate vasogenic oedema, often have cystic component [5, 7–10].

CT findings of gliosarcoma are extremely variable: hyperattenuation in the solid component corresponds to the viable tumour portion and fibrous component, hypoattenuation is typical of the central necrosis. On post-contrast CT scans, gliosarcoma reveals thick, peripheral ring enhancement [7]. Tumour calcification is described in the literature and possibly correspond to chondroid or osteoid metaplasia.

On MRI, gliosarcomas have variable and heterogeneous T1W and T2W signal intensity: generally are hypointense on T1WI, hyper-, iso- or hypointense on T2WI compared to the white matter, and hyperintense on FLAIR. Areas of hyperintensity on T2WI represent gliomatous component with associated necrotic or cystic changes. Hypointense signal of the sarcomatous component on T2WI is due to the dense cellularity and fibrous nature of this non-glial tissue. Due to hypercellularity, solid part of a tumour demonstrates hyperintense signal on DWI and hypointense signal on ADC compatible with diffusion restriction [5, 7–10]. On SWI or T2* sequences areas of variable magnetic susceptibility demonstrate hypointensity within the tumour and may correlate with bleeding or newly formed vessels [7, 11].

After contrast medium administration, gliosarcomas reveal homogeneous or inhomogeneous appearance with thick walls and rim or ring-like contrast enhancement peripheral to necrotic centre [5, 7–10]. On MR spectroscopy lipid and lactate peaks, increased choline and creatine levels are demonstrated [7]. MR perfusion in gliosarcoma shows increased relative cerebral blood volume (rCBV) in tumour and peritumoral regions [5, 7–9].

Gliosarcoma can invade meninges and skull base and can demonstrate extracranial metastases reported in up to 11% of gliosarcoma [12]. Most extracranial metastases of gliosarcoma are located in the lung and liver. There are reports of metastatic foci in cervical lymph nodes, spleen, adrenal glands, kidneys, oral mucosa, skin, bone marrow, skull, ribs and spine. Intramedullary metastasis to the cervical spine has also been reported [13]. According to reports in the literature, metastatic foci consist of biphasic elements or exclusively of sarcomatous component, which points to the sarcomatous component as the potential metastatic source by haematogenous spreading [8, 13].

Two characteristic that may allow to differentiate gliosarcoma from glioblastoma have been described in the literature: the presence of predominantly necrotic lesions associated with nodular thickening at the site of dural attachment, and the presence of predominantly solid lesions [5, 7].

The pathologist remains the final arbiter: diagnosis of gliosarcoma have to be confirmed by histopathological examination. The histopathological criteria that define GSM consist of the detection of a biphasic tumour with two distinct populations of malignant cells, namely glial cells with an astrocytic and anaplastic appearance that fulfil the criteria for GBM; and highly variably mesenchymal cells represented mainly by a fibrosarcomatous component [14]. Immunohistochemically, glial and sarcomatous components can also be differentiated by their expression of glial fibrillary acidic protein (GFAP), that is frequent in the glial component and absent in the sarcomatous component. Another important marker is reticulin, typically present in sarcomatous components. Thus, glial components are typically GFAP-positive and reticulin-negative, whereas the opposite is true for sarcomatous components, i.e. GFAP-negative and reticulin-positive [15].

Gliosarcoma is universally associated with wild-type IDH: the IDH1 mutation is a rare event in this tumour [5, 7].

Differential diagnosis of gliosarcoma includes glioblastoma multiforme and metastasis.

Gliosarcomas have poor prognosis, with a median survival in untreated patients of 4 months and from 6.25 to 11.5 months in treated patients [8]. There is no specific treatment for gliosarcoma which is usually treated using the same therapeutic strategy as for glioblastoma: surgical resection followed by chemotherapy, usually temozolomide, and radiotherapy. Compared with glioblastoma, at surgery gliosarcoma borders are more distinct because of presence of sarcomatous component, but on the other hand, patients have less response to adjuvant treatment including chemotherapy and radiotherapy during postoperative period [16].

Our patient was a male in the seventh decade of his life with symptoms which are in accordance with the tumour location in the left precentral gyrus. Tumour was mainly cystic, had peripheral location in the gyrus with intramural nodule abutting dura. Perilesional vasogenic oedema was mild. Glioblastoma multiforme is a primary brain tumour that reveals many imaging feature. Described imaging features of patient tumour in precentral gyrus could fit the diagnosis of both glioblastoma multiforme and its variant primary gliosarcoma, but metastasis as well. Chest and abdomen CT were performant in the course of diagnostic work-up and did not show primary tumour that could give such metastasis in the precentral gyrus. Cystic form of the tumour, its peripheral location in the precentral gyrus and dural abutment with enhancing nodule at the site of abutment could have point to a specific and rare histopathology of the tumour. In general, it is not possible to differentiate glioblastoma and gliosarcoma only on CT and MR imaging characteristics. Hence, neuroradiologist differential diagnosis for this tumour was correct. Pathologist confirmed diagnosis of gliosarcoma. Most information regarding gliosarcoma published in the literature are case reports with or without review of the literature and review articles regarding epidemiology, imaging, histopathology and treatment of gliosarcoma. We hope we have made a contribution with this case as well.

References

1. Louis DN, et al. The 2016 World Health Organization classification of tumors of the central nervous system: a summary. Acta Neuropathol. 2016;131:803–20.
2. Lutterbacha J, et al. Gliosarcoma: a clinical study. Radiother Oncol. 2001;61(1):57–64.
3. Stroebe H. Ueber Entstehung und Bau der Gehirngliome. Beitr Pathol Mat Allg Pathol. 1895;18:405–86.
4. Feigin I, Gross SW. Sarcoma arising in glioblastoma of the brain. Am J Pathol. 1955;51:633–53.
5. Peckham ME, et al. Gliosarcoma: neuroimaging and immunohistochemical findings. J Neuroimaging. 2019;29(1):126–32.
6. Lucena RCG, et al. Correlação clínico-topográfica em glioblastomas multiformes nas síndromes motoras. Arq Neuropsiquiatr. 2006;64(2-B):441–5.
7. Fukuda A, et al. Gliosarcomas: magnetic resonance imaging findings. Arq Neuropsiquiatr. 2020;78(2):112–20.
8. Sampaio L, et al. Detailed magnetic resonance imaging features of a case series of primary gliosarcoma. Neuroradiol J. 2017;30(6):546–53.
9. Yi X, et al. Gliosarcoma: a clinical and radiological analysis of 48 cases. Eur Radiol. 2018;29(1):429–38.
10. Han L, et al. Magnetic resonance imaging of primary cerebral gliosarcoma: a report of 15 cases. Acta Radiol. 2008;49(9):1058–67.
11. Zhang BY, et al. Computed tomography and magnetic resonance features of gliosarcoma: a study of 54 cases. J Comput Assist Tomogr. 2011;35:667–73.
12. Frandsen S, et al. Clinical characteristics of gliosarcoma and outcomes from standardized treatment relative to conventional glioblastoma. Front Oncol. 2019;9:1425.
13. Han SJ, et al. Primary gliosarcoma: key clinical and pathological distinctions from glioblastoma with implications as a unique oncologic entity. J Neuro-Oncol. 2010;96:312–20.
14. Eisenhauer EA, et al. New response evaluation criteria in solid tumours: revised RECIST guideline (version 1.1). Eur J Cancer. 2009;45(2):228–47.
15. Huo Z, et al. Primary gliosarcoma with long-survival: report of two cases and review of literature. Int J Clin Exp Pathol. 2014;7(9):6323–32.
16. Tabibkhooei A, et al. Gliosarcoma with long progression free survival: a case report and literature review. Surg Neurol Int. 2018;9:227.

A mild right-sided weakness, dysphasia and disorientation were the reason this 80-year-old man was admitted to a neurology department in a local county hospital. He did not have a history of neurologic deficits. Brain CT at the time of admission reported multiple, most likely secondary tumours in the left cerebral hemisphere (Fig. 21.1).

Laboratory and body imaging work-up did not discover evidence of a remote primary neoplastic process. The patient was transferred to our hospital for brain MRI (Fig. 21.2) and neurosurgical work-up.

The patient underwent a robot-assisted stereotactic brain biopsy under neuronavigation, which was uneventful. The patient remained neurologically stable. A CT exam of the brain performed several hours post surgery (Fig. 21.3a, b) demonstrated intracerebral and subarachnoid bleed in the biopsy bed. The patient was treated conservatively, and there was no evidence of haematoma progression in the next follow-up CT exam performed 8 h later (Fig. 21.3c, d).

Several days later, the histopathology report was ready: it stated thick areas of atypical astroglial cells with marked polymorphism and mitotic activity (Ki67: 15%), evidence of focal necrosis, GFAP positive, IDH-1 negative—findings consistent with a glioblastoma (WHO grade IV).

21.1 Glioblastoma

Glioblastoma (GB), previously known as glioblastoma multiforme, is the most common malignant primary brain tumour in adults. It accounts for approximately 48% of all primary malignant CNS tumours, representing approximately 57% of all gliomas. It affects men more frequently than women (1.58:1) with a highest incidence in Caucasians, somewhat lower in Asians and significantly lower incidence in people of African descent (1.93:1). The median age at diagnosis is 65 years, but incidence is the highest in patients aged 75–84 years [1, 2]. For the less frequent IDH-mutant ("IDH positive")-type glioblastoma (see below), the median age is 44 years, and the prognosis is somewhat better. Generally, glioblastoma diagnosis bears a poor prognosis, with overall 5-year survival being only 5.8% [2].

There are few risk factors associated with glioblastoma, the strongest being exposure to ionizing radiation [1–3], mostly during radiation therapy (RT) for other neoplasms. The median administered RT dose in a research by Elsamadicy et al. [3] was 35.6 Gy, but the most common dosage was between 21–30 Gy and 41–50 Gy. The median latency period between RT and development of radiation-induced malignant glioma (RIMG) was 9 years. In 82%

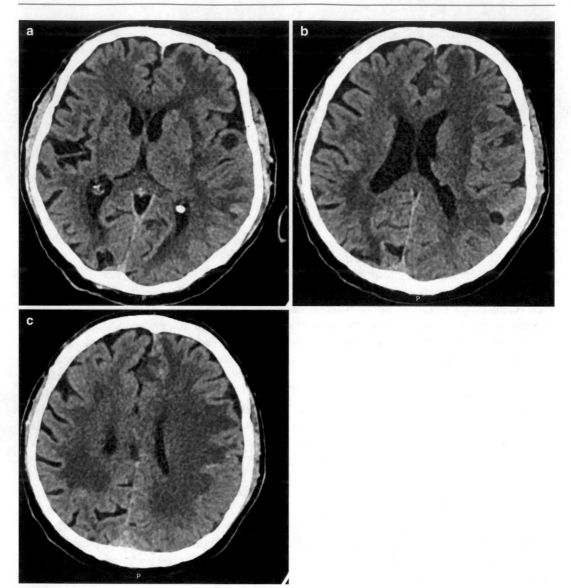

Fig. 21.1 Non-enhanced CT exam of the brain. Cystic-appearing lesions in the left frontoparietal operculum, without appreciable perifocal oedema (**a**, **b**). Disruption of the normal parenchymal structure at the grey–white matter junction in the left rostral medial frontal region (**c**)

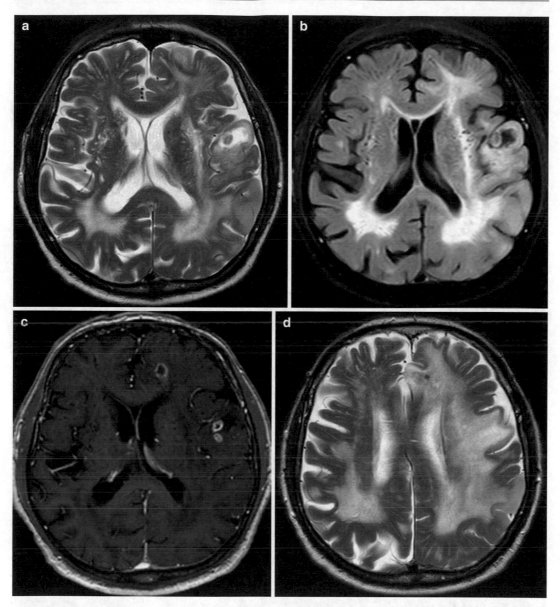

Fig. 21.2 MRI exam of the brain with MR spectroscopy. Axial T2WI (**a**, **d**), axial T2-FLAIR (**b**, **e**), axial contrast-enhanced T1WI (**c**, **f**), coronal T2WI (**g**), axial DWI (**h**) and ADC map (**i**), single-voxel MR spectroscopy (TE 144 ms) (**j**). Left frontal, mostly subcortical rim-enhancing lesions with internal low diffusion; perifocal vasogenic oedema. Single-voxel spectroscopy (SVS) of the largest peripherally enhanced lesion demonstrates elevated choline and creatine levels with a lactate peak (inverted). Report conclusion suggested an inflammatory/infectious aetiology, with cerebritis and multiple abscesses

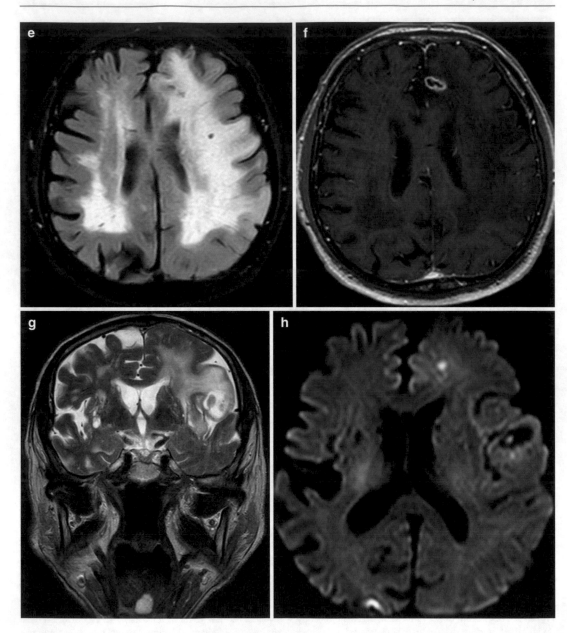

Fig. 21.2 (continued)

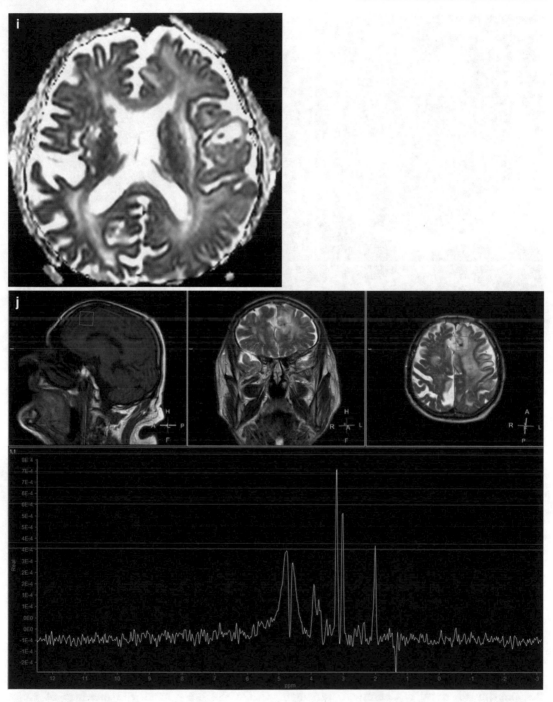

Fig. 21.2 (continued)

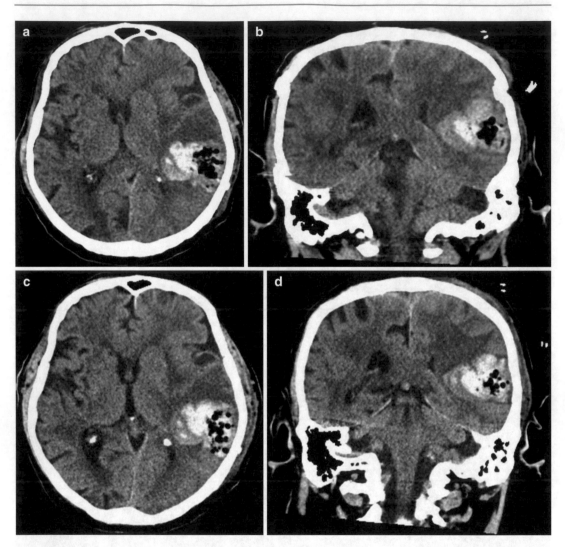

Fig. 21.3 First (**a**, **b**) and second (**c**, **d**) post-biopsy CT exam of the brain. There is a haematoma in the biopsy bed, representing a biopsy complication

of patients RIMG occurred within 15 years from RT. Children, especially under 5 years of age, are at greater risk for RIMG developing later in life [4]. There also appears to be a statistically significant increase in the incidence of brain malignancies in cleanup workers after the nuclear disaster in Chernobyl, although their average radiation dose was relatively low (0.1 Gy) [4]. RIMG do not feature specific histologic or molecular features.

Some rare genetic syndromes are associated with glioblastoma, such as Li-Fraumeni syndrome and Lynch syndrome, but they account

for less than 1% of cases [1, 2]. There is also the ever-lingering theory of mobile phones increasing risk for brain tumours, but this has not been established for gliomas in adults (although there seems to be a positive correlation with acoustic neuroma occurrence) [5].

On the other hand, the presence of atopy, allergies and other immune-related conditions appears to be associated with a lower incidence of glioma (including glioblastoma) [1, 2].

The pathophysiology of gliomagenesis is still unclear. The most favoured theory is the development from neuroglial progenitor cells—

neural stem cells, glial precursor cells and oligodendrocyte precursor cells [1, 2].

The presence or absence of isocitrate-dehydrogenase (IDH) mutation determines the main glioblastoma classification by the WHO. IDH mutation can produce high levels of 2-hydroxyglutaric acid (2-HG), which inhibits stem cell differentiation. At the same time, IDH mutation enables vascular endothelial growth factor (VEGF) to promote the formation of the tumour microenvironment. Additionally, IDH mutation can also produce high levels of hypoxia-inducible factor-1α (HIF-1α) to promote glioma invasion [6]. IDH1 gene is located on the long arm of chromosome 2 (2q32) and encodes for cytosolic isocitrate dehydrogenase, while IDH2 is located on the long arm of chromosome 15 (15q21) and encodes for mitochondrial isocitrate dehydrogenase.

The majority of glioblastomas (approximately 90%) are primary glioblastomas or glioblastoma IDH wild-type (IDH-wt), negative for IDH mutations. They arise de novo from non-neoplastic brain and grow aggressively. A smaller fraction of glioblastomas (up to 10%) are secondary glioblastomas or glioblastomas IDH-mutant (IDH-positive). Secondary glioblastomas arise from a prior lower-grade glioma (e.g. diffuse astrocytoma, anaplastic astrocytoma) and harbour a mutation in IDH-1 or IDH-2 genes which occur early in gliomagenesis. Both the subtypes are high-grade astrocytic tumours with areas of microvascular proliferation and/or focal necrosis. The IDH wild-type glioblastoma is somewhat histologically varied and may contain pleomorphic, multinucleated giant cells (giant cell glioblastoma), sarcoma-like mesenchymal metaplasia (gliosarcoma, see Chap. 20) and more prominent epithelioid morphology (epithelioid glioblastoma) [2].

On the molecular level, approximately 60% of IDH-wt glioblastomas contain over-expressed epidermal growth factor receptors (EGFR) [7], 83% harbour pTERT (telomerase reverse transcriptase promoter) gene mutation and phosphatase and tensin homolog (PTEN) gene deletion. These mutations do not have to occur across the whole tumour volume, but they can be expressed in just one clone of tumour cells forming one region of the glioblastoma. Approximately half of the mutations are regionally exclusive [1, 8]. Only mutation of pTERT gene tends to be already present in the founding clone, i.e. when present, it is harboured in all tumoural cells [8] If occurring as an isolated mutation, it is associated with significantly lower overall survival [8]. On the other hand, promoter methylation at the O^6-methylguanine-DNA-methyltransferase (MGMT) locus seen in 30–50% of IDH-wt glioblastoma brings a more favourable prognosis because it renders the tumour susceptible to alkylating chemotherapy (temozolomide) [2].

Secondary glioblastomas harbour the IDH mutations, but may be distinguished by the presence of ATRX (alpha thalassemia/mental retardation syndrome X-linked, 57% of cases) and TP53 gene (60% of cases) mutations, which are often found in lower-grade gliomas [9].

Except for IDH-wt and IDH-mutant, there is a third subtype of grade IV gliomas added by The World Health Organization classification of CNS tumours in 2016: H3F3A or HIST1H3B/C K27M (H3-K27M)-mutant, diffuse midline glioma, occurring predominantly in children and young adults and bearing a dismal prognosis [2].

The clinical presentations of glioblastomas are varied and depend on the functional aspect of the involved brain parenchyma. Symptoms like speech disturbances, numbness, loss of vision and persistent weakness are often associated with a smaller tumour on initial imaging. Mood disorders, fatigue, mild memory disorders and executive dysfunction tend to be the presentation symptoms of larger tumours involving frontal lobe, temporal lobe or corpus callosum. Seizures occur in 25% of patients with newly diagnosed glioblastoma and are often easy to control with medications [10].

On imaging, glioblastoma is typically hypodense on CT, hyperdense on MRI, with the appearance of an infiltrative, heterogeneous, peripherally enhancing lesion with central necrosis and surrounding vasogenic oedema of variable size, with mass effect. Glioblastoma-produced oedema often extends to the cortex and/or deep grey matter at least along one portion of the lesion and is infiltrative in nature [11], which in practice means that there is tumour infiltration in the T2 hyperdense area beyond the irregular rim of T1 post-contrast enhancement. Multifocal enhancement is uncommon, but there can be smaller satellite areas of enhancement and necrosis—again that often includes tumour infiltration between the areas of enhancement, as well. Rarely the tumour appears as a small non-enhancing or partially enhancing lesion, but it rapidly progresses into a more common form with ring enhancement and necrosis [10]. Large intratumoural haemorrhage is rare, but there are often smaller areas of blood products producing low signal on T2[1] and susceptibility weighted images. The solid portions of the tumour are commonly low in ADC maps which reflects low diffusion, while necrotic portions demonstrate high signal on ADC maps. MR spectroscopy shows increased choline, lactates and lipids and decreased NAA. The hallmark of GBM on perfusion studies is very high rCBV of solid tumour areas [11]. Elevation of rCBV to a lesser extent is seen in the peritumoural zone of the infiltrative oedema [12]. IDH-mutant glioblastoma initially may be non-enhancing, with cortical infiltration and minimal oedema and necrosis, with a predilection for frontal and temporal lobes [2].

Differential diagnoses include:

- Metastasis, which often has a large perifocal vasogenic oedema outside of the enhancing area; the oedema is not infiltrative, and the tissue it involves shows normal values on MR spectroscopy and MR perfusion [11].
- Primary CNS lymphoma, which is rarely necrotic (except in HIV-positive patients), enhances homogenously and shows very low diffusion (hypointense in ADC maps) and prominent vasogenic oedema,
- Cerebral abscess, with a smooth and complete SWI-hypointense rim and low diffusion in the central necrotic part. Dual rim sign in SWI and T2WI is specific (if present—in 75% of cases).

- Tumefactive demyelinating lesion (TDL) (*see footnote 1*), with a characteristic incomplete ring of enhancement and low rCBV on perfusion imaging [11].
- Subacute cerebral infarction (*see footnote 1*), following a vascular territory, with a common gyriform enhancement and a low rCBV, lacking choline elevation on MRS.

The standard initial therapy for glioblastomas in patients younger than 70 years of age is maximal safe surgical resection, although GTR is virtually impossible due to infiltrative tumour growth. Surgery provides reduction of the tumour mass and the tissue for histopathological and molecular analysis. In cases where a large surgery is not indicated or diagnosis is uncertain, biopsy is performed to obtain a tissue sample for analysis and further treatment planning.

The surgery is followed by radiation therapy (60 Gy in 2-Gy fractions over 6 weeks) with concomitant temozolomide (TMZ), and then adjuvant TMZ [1, 2]. Glioblastoma patients with MGMT gene mutation treated with an alkylating agent chemotherapy (e.g. TMZ) have a longer survival than those without MGMT methylation and those treated with radiotherapy alone [1].

Elderly patients aged 70 years and over generally have worse prognosis, many of them are unfit for conventional long-term radiation. A modified RT approach (40 Gy delivered in 2.67-Gy fractions over 3 weeks), especially combined with TMZ where suitable, has proven to be beneficial in terms of overall survival.

Bevacizumab (not approved in Europe for glioblastoma treatment) is a monoclonal antibody (MAB) that inhibits VEGF, thus acting as an antiangiogenic agent, but its results in glioblastoma therapy were not encouraging because of increased toxicity without difference in overall survival [2]. However, some physicians use bevacizumab to reduce the burden of cerebral oedema and spare the patient from high doses of corticosteroids [1].

A locoregional therapy by tumour-treating fields (TTFs) is approved as an adjuvant ther-

---

[1]As explained in our previous book *Neuroradiology: Expect the Unexpected.*

apy in combination with TMZ. It consists of four transducer arrays connected to a portable device generating low-intensity, alternating electric fields of 200 Hz which suppress normal tumour cell division. The arrays are applied to the shaved scalp for at least 18 h a day [1, 2]. The feedback proved good compliance and mild to moderate cutaneous toxicity typically resolved with minimal intervention [1]. TTFs are applied with maintenance therapy of temozolomide, after the end of initial 6 week chemoradiotherapy, and the patients receiving them with TMZ fared better than patients treated with TMZ alone [1].

There are some novel therapies being tested, such as intratumoural injection of oncolytic viruses and chimeric antigen receptor (CAR)-modified T-cells [1, 2].

Supportive therapy includes an array of different medications: antiepileptic therapy controls seizures which occur in 80% of patients during the course of disease; vasogenic oedema is treated with corticosteroids; venous thromboembolism prophylaxis with low-molecular-weight heparin should start 24 h after surgery; lymphopenia caused by temozolomide, corticosteroids and radiotherapy may give rise to opportunistic infections by *Pneumocystis jiroveci* (previously known as *Pneumocystis carinii*) which may be prevented by antibiotic prophylaxis [2].

References

1. Lukas RV, et al. Newly diagnosed glioblastoma: a review on clinical management. Oncology (Williston Park). 2019;33(3):91–100.

2. Tan AC, et al. Management of glioblastoma: state of the art and future directions. CA Cancer J Clin. 2020;70(4):299–312. https://doi.org/10.3322/caac.21613.

3. Elsamadicy AA, et al. Radiation-induced malignant gliomas: a current review. World Neurosurg. 2015;83(4):530–42. https://doi.org/10.1016/j.wneu.2014.12.009.

4. Prasad G, Haas-Kogan DA. Radiation-induced gliomas. Expert Rev Neurother. 2009;9(10):1511–7. https://doi.org/10.1002/pmic.200800802.

5. Vienne-Jumeau A, et al. Environmental risk factors of primary brain tumors: a review. Rev Neurol. 2019;175(10):664–78. https://doi.org/10.1016/j.neurol.2019.08.004.

6. Huang J, et al. Isocitrate dehydrogenase mutations in glioma: from basic discovery to therapeutics development. Front Oncol. 2019;9(506):12. https://doi.org/10.3389/fonc.2019.00506.

7. Xu H, et al. Epidermal growth factor receptor in glioblastoma. Oncol Lett. 2017;14(1):512–6. https://doi.org/10.3892/ol.2017.6221.

8. Mahlokozera T, et al. Biological and therapeutic implications of multisector sequencing in newly diagnosed glioblastoma. Neuro-Oncology. 2018;20(4):472–83. https://doi.org/10.1093/neuonc/nox232.

9. Chaurasia A, et al. Immunohistochemical analysis of ATRX, IDH1 and p53 in glioblastoma and their correlations with patient survival. J Korean Med Sci. 2016;31(8):1208–14. https://doi.org/10.3346/jkms.2016.31.8.1208.

10. Alexander BM, Cloughesy TF. Adult glioblastoma. J Clin Oncol Off J Am Soc Clin Oncol. 2017;35(21):2402–9. https://doi.org/10.1200/JCO.2017.73.0119.

11. Rumboldt Z. Glioblastoma multiforme. In: Brain imaging with MRI and CT: an image pattern approach. Cambridge University Press; 2012. p. 316–7.

12. Neska-Matuszewska M, et al. Differentiation of glioblastoma multiforme, metastases and primary central nervous system lymphomas using multiparametric perfusion and diffusion MR imaging of a tumor core and a peritumoral zone-searching for a practical approach. PLoS One. 2018;13(1):e0191341. https://doi.org/10.1371/journal.pone.0191341.

Extradural Spinal Meningioma

After a month of persisting low back pain and bilateral leg weakness, this 55-year-old woman sought help at our Emergency Hospital Department, where upon clinical examination spastic paraparesis was diagnosed. Two weeks prior, she had had a lumbar spine MRI done in another institution which revealed degenerative stenosis with bilateral L4 and right-sided L5 and S1 spinal nerve root compressions. However, these could not explain the severity of the neurological symptoms, including sensory disturbance at T10 level and below. She was admitted to the neurology department where a comprehensive workup was initiated.

The blood tests were unremarkable. The patient had no other health problems.

A thoracic spine MRI exam was performed, showing a lesion within the spinal canal (Fig. 22.1).

The initial impression of an enhancing lesion almost wrapped around the spinal cord, with cord compression and myelopathy, was suspicious of lymphoproliferative infiltration. However, the detailed cytology studies of the CSF and blood did not support that diagnosis. Finally, neurosurgeons decided they would try to remove the lesion—laminectomy was performed in segments T6–T8, and the epidural mass was resected. There was an inadvertent lesion of the dura 30 mm in length which was repaired immediately. The patient's recovery was uneventful, very soon she started to recover her ability to walk.

Histopathology reported the resected mass to be a meningioma (WHO grade I).

Three months later, follow-up MRI (Fig. 22.2) reported a small residual tumour, which did not change in another 3- month interval. The patient reported occasional tingling in her legs, but no other symptoms.

22.1 Extradural Spinal Meningioma (ESM)

Meningiomas are the second most common tumours occurring in the spinal canal, after schwannomas—they account for approximately 25% of tumours in this location [1]. However, they make only 1.2% of all CNS meningiomas [2]. The majority of spinal meningiomas are intradural extramedullary, while only 2.5–3.5% [3] of them are extradural (epidural)—thus, the ESMs make a mere 0.03% of all CNS meningiomas. The small number of reported cases of ESM and varied criteria to differentiate between completely and partially extradural meningiomas do not provide for precise statistics; there seems to be a predilection for patients in their fourth decade of life, with women being somewhat more often affected than men [1, 3, 4]. The most common location is thoracic spine, followed by cervical and lumbar spine [2, 4].

These tumours may originate from remnants of the arachnoid cap cells at the exiting nerve root

M. Špero, H. Vavro, *Neuroradiology - Images vs Symptoms*,
https://doi.org/10.1007/978-3-030-69213-1_22

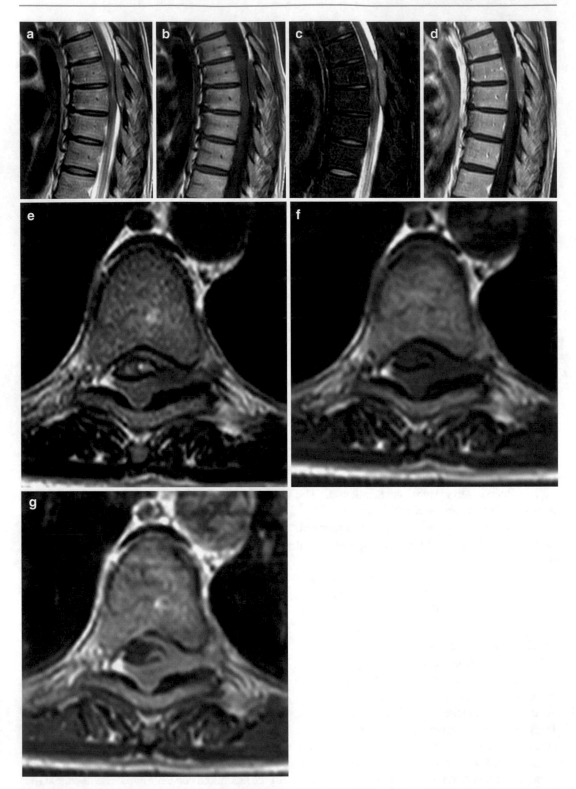

Fig. 22.1 MRI of the thoracic spine. Sagittal T2WI (**a**), sagittal T1WI (**b**), sagittal STIR image (**c**), sagittal contrast-enhanced T1WI (**d**), axial T2WI (**e**), axial T1WI (**f**), axial contrast-enhanced T1WI (**g**). In segments T7 and T8, there is a solid, moderately enhancing extradural lesion in the left, anterior and posterior aspects of the spinal canal, compressing the spinal cord (half-ring shape, see below) and extending into the left neural foramen. Signs of compression myelopathy—note a small area of cord enhancement due to myelopathy on the left

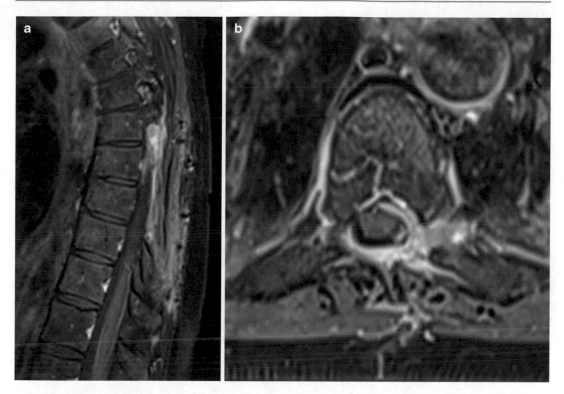

Fig. 22.2 Follow-up MRI of the thoracic spine 5 months after surgery, contrast-enhanced sagittal (**a**) and axial (**b**) fat suppressed T1WI. There is an enhancing small resid- ual meningioma in the left and posterior aspects of the spinal canal, extending into the left neural foramen T7–T8 but without spinal cord compression

sheath or elsewhere in the epidural space, or from the vertebral periosteum [1, 4]. The large majority of them are WHO grade I. The ESMs tend to grow more aggressively than their intradural counterparts, which is mirrored by relatively rapid neurological decline (symptoms depending on the affected spinal level) and invasive features on imaging, e.g. infiltration of the dura and the adjacent soft tissues [4] including nerve roots [1] and bony erosion and remodelling of the adjacent vertebral arch and pedicle. These imaging fea- tures are the reason they often get misdiagnosed as metastases, especially if the patient has a his- tory of a malignant disease.

The most frequent presenting symptom is pain, followed by sensory and motor deficits, depending on the affected spinal cord segment and nerve root.

On imaging, MRI typically demonstrates a dumbbell-shaped (possibly extending through the neural foramen), ovoid or en plaque tumour narrowing the spinal canal, isointense in T1WI,

iso- or hypointense in T2WI, with homogenous contrast enhancement, almost always with a "dural tail" [1]. The diffusion in DWI/ADC maps may be compromised [4]. En plaque ESMs often have a half-ring appearance to them on axial images. CT may demonstrate calcification which could be a telltale for meningioma diagnosis and it appears to be more common than in intradural meningiomas [1]. There are suggestions that cal- cified meningiomas are prone to recurring which may also be related to more difficult complete removal of such tumours.

Differential diagnoses include lymphomas which are often T2WI hypointense and diffusion- restricting and appear mostly in the ventral dura forming a paravertebral mass and infiltrating the adjacent bone (unlike ESMs which tend to erode or compress the bone rather than infiltrate it). Other extradural tumours tend to be hyperintense in T2WI. Dumbbell-shaped ESMs differ from neurogenic tumours (e.g. schwannoma, neurofi- broma) by homogenous enhancement and calcification. Metastatic tumours often cause adjacent bone destruction and paravertebral tissue involvement. Posterior longitudinal ligament ossification does not demonstrate dural enhancement nor thickening [1].

Treatment consists of GTR (gross total resection). As ESMs are sometimes confused with metastases, initial palliative surgical approach may be extended into a GTR after a histopathological confirmation of a meningioma. Therefore, intraoperative histology is mandatory [4]. Recurrence is fairly common, mostly due to resection difficulties caused by adherence of the tumour to the dura or the nerve roots or invasion of the adjacent soft tissues. Calcified tumours are more difficult to resect and recur more often. Long-term follow-up is important, as the longest recurrence interval reported was 192 months (16 years).

References

1. Zhang LH, Yuan HS. Imaging appearances and pathologic characteristics of spinal epidural meningioma. AJNR Am J Neuroradiol. 2018;39(1):199–204. https://doi.org/10.3174/ajnr.A5414.
2. Sandalcioglu IE, et al. Spinal meningiomas: critical review of 131 surgically treated patients. Eur Spine J. 2008;17(8):1035–41. https://doi.org/10.1007/s00586-008-0685-y.
3. Dehcordi SR, et al. Dorsal extradural meningioma: case report and literature review. Surg Neurol Int. 2016;7:76. https://doi.org/10.4103/2152-7806.188914.
4. Lai AL, et al. Extradural cervical spinal meningioma mimicking malignancy. J Radiol Case Rep. 2018;12(10):1–10. https://doi.org/10.3941/jrcr.v12i10.3498.

Chronic Venous Sinus Thrombosis vs Brain Metastases

In November 2018, a 72-year-old female patient presented with sudden onset of dysarthria followed by short-term spasm of right hemifacial spasm. She had a history of arterial hypertension, diabetes and hyperlipidaemia. There was no evidence of head trauma or loss of consciousness.

On admission, C-reactive protein, blood count, prothrombin time, blood glucose and electrolytes were within normal range, urea and creatinine were slightly elevated. Blood pressure was elevated, 180/100 mm Hg, she was afebrile. Brain CT was performed in the EHD: small subcortical intracerebral haematoma in the left frontal lobe was reported (Fig. 23.1).

Due to CT finding of intracerebral haematoma, the patient was hospitalized. Symptoms did not improve on applied therapy, and 7 days later, MRI of the brain was performed (Figs. 23.2 and 23.3).

Analysing brain MRI (Figs. 23.2 and 23.3), neuroradiologist reported intracerebral haematoma in the left inferior frontal gyrus not typical for a primary intracerebral haematoma (Figs. 23.2a–d, h). Small subcortical contras enhancing lesion within the vasogenic oedema in the left middle temporal gyrus was understood as a possible small metastasis (Fig. 23.2e, f, i). In the same context, intracerebral haematoma in the left inferior frontal gyrus was considered to be a haemorrhagic metastasis as well. Dilated cortical vein with dilated deep medullary veins was misunderstood as possible prominent developmental venous anomaly (Figs. 23.2g and 23.3). There was no evidence of arteriovenous malformation or fistula. As a less obvious differential diagnosis primary brain lymphoma with perivascular infiltration was mentioned.

In further diagnostic work-up body CT did not reveal primary tumour that would give brain metastases. Further, left temporal bone trepanation and robot-assisted stereotactic biopsy of the enhancing lesion in the left middle temporal gyrus was performed. Final pathologist report was gliotic tissue without elements of a tumour growth for the first cylinder of tissue and granulation tissue with erythrocyte and siderophage extravasation for the second cylinder of tissue.

Pathologist report indicated necessity for a revision of MRI study. After a second look, diagnosis of thrombosis of the anterior part of the superior sagittal sinus was made resulting in the development of significant collateral drainage through the parenchymal veins and dilatation of adjoining cortical cerebral vein which was thrombosed as well. Thrombosis of the superior sagittal sinus was understood as chronic due to signal intensities: there was

M. Špero, H. Vavro, *Neuroradiology - Images vs Symptoms*,
https://doi.org/10.1007/978-3-030-69213-1_23

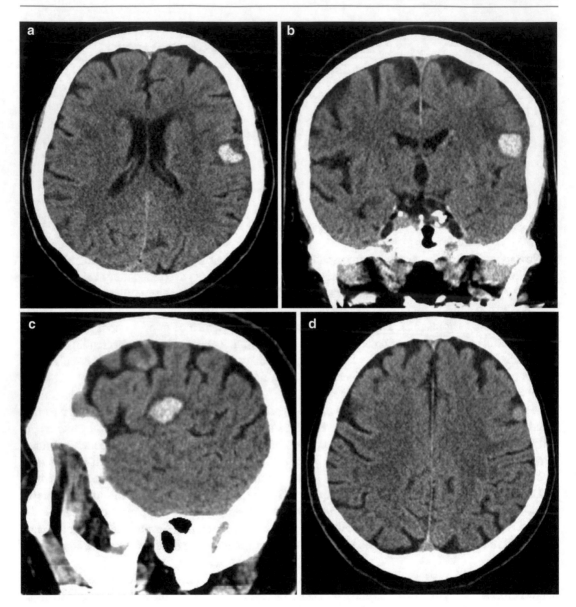

Fig. 23.1 Computed tomography of the brain, non-contrast axial (**a**, **d**), coronal (**b**, **e**), and sagittal (**c**, **f**), revealed small subcortical intracerebral haematoma in the left inferior frontal gyrus, measuring 14 × 16 × 12 mm, surrounded by a mild vasogenic oedema (**a–c**). Small, oval extra-axial hyperdense lesion adjacent to left middle frontal gyrus presenting thrombosed, dilated cortical vein (**d–f**), was not reported by radiologist on call

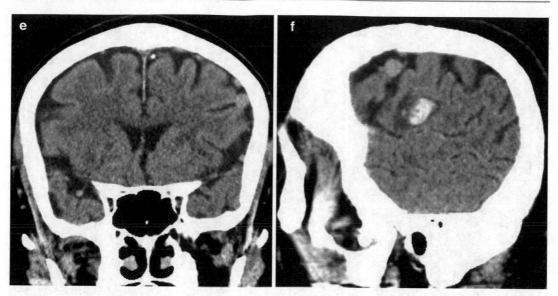

Fig. 23.1 (continued)

no evidence of flow void on T2WI (Fig. 23.3b, c) and no evidence of flow within the sinus on MRV (Fig. 23.3d–f) which was hyperintense on T2WI (Fig. 23.3b, c). Contrast in the sinus without intraluminal filling defect on T1 MPRAGE indicated intrinsic vascularization in organized thrombus within the sinus lumen (Fig. 23.3g–i). Chronic venous thrombosis resulted in secondary haemorrhagic infarcts which were misunderstood as haemorrhagic metastases.

Afterwards, acetylsalicylic acid was introduced in therapy. On follow-up MRI, cortical vein on the surface of the left frontal lobe was not dilated, there was no contrast in the vessel lumen and no evidence of a flow within the vein on MRV (Fig. 23.4).

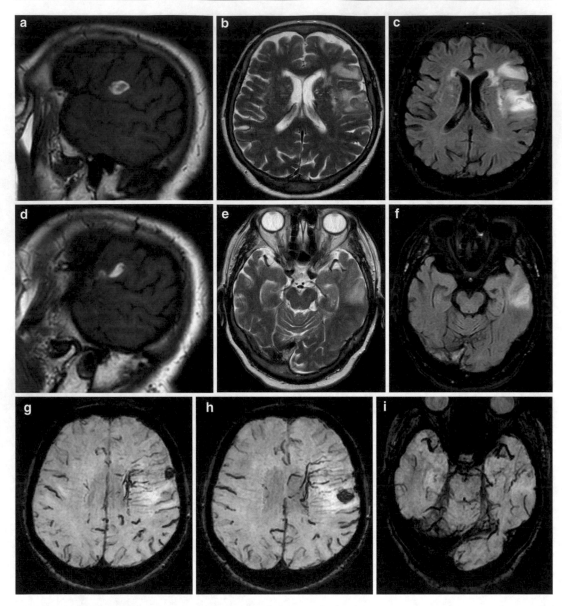

Fig. 23.2 Magnetic resonance imaging of the brain, non-contrast, sagittal T1WI (**a**, **d**), axial T2WI (**b**, **e**), FLAIR FS (**c**, **f**), SWI (**g**–**i**), in comparison to head CT confirmed subcortical intracerebral haematoma in the left inferior frontal gyrus, surrounding vasogenic oedema was progressed involving frontal operculum, insula and anterior part of the superior and medial temporal gyrus with narrow adjacent sulci. On axial SWI (**i**), there were few sub-cortical punctiforme hypointensities in the medial temporal gyrus with punctiforme hyperintensity on T1WI (**a**). Cortical cerebral vein adjacent to the left middle frontal gyrus was dilated and markedly hypointense on SWI revealing "blooming effect" (**g**) while deep medullary veins in the parenchyma of the left frontal lobe were prominent showing flow voids on SWI (**g**, **h**)

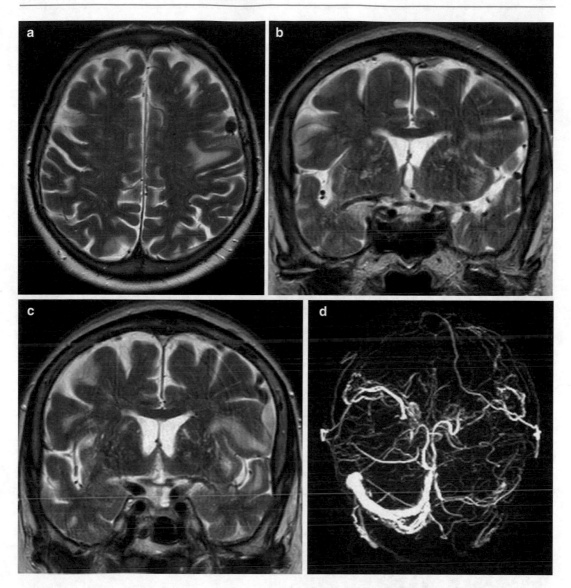

Fig. 23.3 Magnetic resonance imaging of the brain, T2WI coronal (**a**) and axial (**b**, **c**), post-contrast T1 MPRAGE axial (**g**, **h**) and coronal (**i**), MR venography (3D PC technique) axial (**d**), coronal (**e**), sagittal (**f**). Dilated cortical cerebral vein adjacent to the left middle frontal gyrus was hypointense on T2WI, without evidence of flow through the vein on MRV. There was no evidence of contrast in the vein on post-contrast T1 MPRAGE (**g**). Anterior part of the superior sagittal sinus was hyperintense on T2WI: there was no flow through it on MRV, while on post-contrast T1 MPRAGE sequence it showed contrast in the sinus, without intraluminal filling defect. On post-contrast T1 MPRAGE deep medullary veins in the left inferior and middle frontal gyrus were prominent, "squiggly" while traversing parenchyma towards the ventricular wall. There was small subcortical nodular contrast enhancement within vasogenic oedema involving the anterior part of the middle temporal gyrus

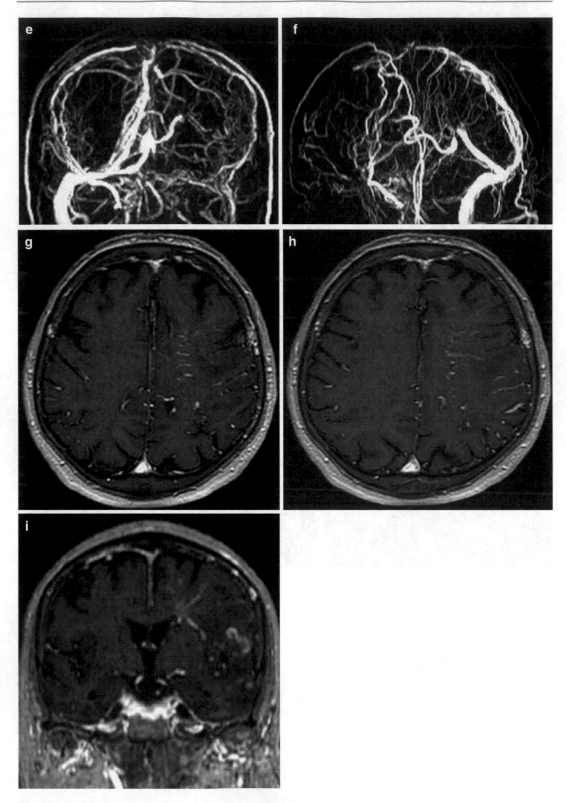

Fig. 23.3 (continued)

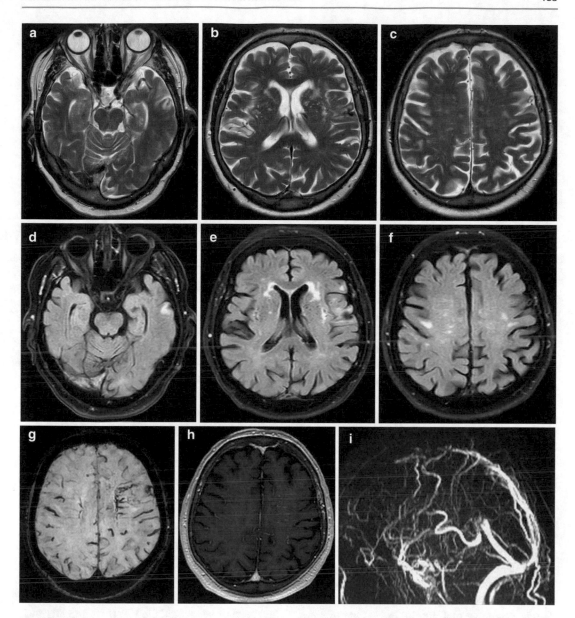

Fig. 23.4 Follow-up magnetic resonance imaging of the brain, non-contrast axial T2WI (**a–c**), FLAIR FS (**d–f**), SWI (**g**), post-contrast T1 MPRAGE (**h**), sagittal MRV (**i**). Venous infarcts in the left frontal and temporal lobes have regressed, gliosis developed, deep medullary veins in the frontal lobe were still prominent, anterior part of the supe-rior sagittal sinus was thrombosed demonstrating contrast enhancement. Cortical vein on the surface of the left fron-tal lobe was not dilated any more, there was no contrast in the vessel lumen and no evidence of a flow within the vein on MRV: its content was hypointense on FLAIR and hyperintense on T2WI

23.1 Chronic Venous Sinus Thrombosis vs Brain Metastases

Cerebral venous sinus thrombosis (CVST) is not uncommon vascular disorder. It develops due to thrombus of dural venous sinus causing an acute neurological deterioration with possible fatal outcome if not diagnosed in early stage.

CVST can occur at any age: it is more common in neonates and young adults between 20 and 40 years old, especially in women of reproductive age due to pregnancy, postpartum status, and use of oral contraceptives [1]. It is responsible for 1–2% of stroke in these group of patients [2].

According to recently published data, annual incidence of CVST is three or four to 13 cases per one million individuals [3–5]. The differences in incidence in conducted studies are likely due to differences in diagnostic techniques [1]. The incidence varies in different parts of the world, being higher in Asia, the Middle East and Africa, probably due to a higher occurrence of known risk factors [2]. Known risk factors and causes of CVST are venous thromboembolism, pregnancy, oestrogen therapy/oral contraceptives, thrombophilia (especially antithrombin deficiency, protein C and S deficiency and factor V Leiden mutation), hypercoagulability as part of inflammatory disease, head trauma (skull fracture extending to the dural sinus or the jugular bulb is associated with sinus thrombosis), local infections and underlying cancer. In general, the most common predisposing factor for this condition is hypercoagulability in the context of a prothrombotic condition, but up to 20% of cases are idiopathic, so the absence of risk factors does not rule out the diagnosis [1].

Obstruction due to dural sinus or cortical vein thrombosis results in an increased venous pressure and reduced capillary perfusion. At first, an increase in retrograde venous pressure leads to venous congestion and drainage through the cerebral collateral vessels which are dilated. Outbalanced capacity of collateral vessels results in venous stasis, increased intramural pressure and damage to veins and the blood–brain barrier.

Those changes manifests with vasogenic oedema and haemorrhagic infarcts. Reduction in cerebral perfusion leads to cytotoxic oedema and reduced absorption of cerebrospinal fluid that further increases intracranial pressure [1, 2].

Clinical diagnosis of CSVT is difficult to make because patients present with a wide spectrum of non-specific symptoms also seen in more common diagnoses, like stroke or brain tumours. Most common presenting symptoms are headache, followed by focal neurological deficits, seizures or decreased level of consciousness, which occur in the setting of focal or diffuse cerebral oedema, venous non-haemorrhagic or haemorrhagic infarct. Imaging procedures, CT and MRI should confirm diagnosis of CSVT.

Symptom onset may be acute, subacute or chronic. Due to a slow growth of thrombus and extensive venous collateralization, symptoms typically evolve over days or weeks with subacute onset, although the onset may be acute and chronic as well. The severity of symptoms depends on chronicity of development and on the vessels involved [6].

Cerebral venous sinus thrombosis should be suspected in a case of progressive headache or other symptoms that raise suspicion of the condition in the setting of known predisposing factors. No specific laboratory tests confirm the diagnosis: elevated D-dimer level may support the diagnosis, but a normal level is not sufficient to rule out the condition [7]. Head CT is fast and widely available imaging method, therefore is usually the initial imaging procedure in the EHD in a case of suspected CSVT. If technically possible, MRI could be performed as the first-line imaging procedure. CT and MRI provide insight into whether there is evidence of direct or indirect signs of CSVT and exclude other causes of presenting symptoms, such as stroke, subarachnoid haemorrhage or brain tumour. CT venography (CTV) and MR venography (MRV) should be performed as a part of CT or MRI brain investigations to confirm diagnosis. However, in more than 30% of cases, neither direct nor indirect signs of cerebral venous thrombosis are seen on CT scans [2], and MRI of the brain and MR venography provide superior visualisation of the brain parenchyma, venous infarcts and haemorrhages, thus are preferred imaging modalities. Technique of choice for diagnostic evaluation and follow-up of dural sinus thrombosis is MR venography [6].

The cohort study on cerebral venous thrombosis by Ferro et al. showed that cerebral venous thrombosis involves venous system in descending frequency: superior sagittal sinus (62%), left and right transverse sinus (44.7% and 41.2%, respectively), straight sinus (18%), cortical veins (17.1%), deep venous system (10.9%), cavernous sinus (1.3%), and cerebellar veins (0.3%) [8].

Direct imaging signs of CVST indicate the presence of thrombus in the affected venous sinus or vein. According to the literature, direct signs include cord sign, dense triangle sing and empty delta or empty triangle sign. "Cord sign" represents elongated hyper-attenuating acute thrombus within a vein. "Dense triangle sign" corresponds to a fresh thrombus in the venous sinus. These signs are identified on noncontrast CT in acute phase, but may persist for up to 2 weeks, after which thrombus becomes isodense to brain parenchyma. They are nonspecific because slow flow can produce it, or may be visible in patients with raised haematocrit or dehydration [9, 10]. On CT venography, contrast media surrounds thrombus, making it clearly visible as a filling defect which is the most frequent sign of thrombosis named "empty triangle sign" or "empty delta sign" when the torcular herophili or superior sagittal sinus is involved. The empty delta sign is seen in 29%–35% of cases and may be absent in the acute phases of the process, in which the thrombus is hyperattenuating (mimicking opacification of the sinus), and in the chronic phases, in which the thrombus can contain recanalization channels [1].

MRI is more sensitive for revealing thrombus due to combination of sequences and high sensitivity to the magnetic susceptibility of blood degradation products, notably on gradient echo T2-weighted images (T2*). The signal intensity of venous thrombi on T1WI and T2WI depend on the interval between the onset of thrombus formation and the time of imaging due to the para-

magnetic effects of haemoglobin degradation products [1]. In early or acute stages (<5 days), thrombus appears isointense on T1WI and hypointense on T2WI due to oxyhaemoglobin and deoxyhaemoglobin stage, thus almost mimicking the normal venous flow signal and creating a potential for diagnostic error. Evaluation with a contrast-enhanced CT or MRI is thus essential at this stage to confidently rule out thrombosis [9, 10]. In subacute phase (5–30 days) due to methaemoglobin content thrombus is hyperintense on both T1WI and T2WI. During chronic stages, the presentation pattern in the MRI is more variable. The thrombosed venous sinus can recanalize itself or remain either partially or completely occluded, which can be interpreted as a recurrent CVT [11]. Chronic thrombosis with incomplete recanalization of the sinus may present a diagnostic challenge at MR imaging. About 15% of patients with diagnosed venous sinus thrombosis may have a chronic thrombus on MRI. Compared with the MR signal in normal brain parenchyma, the signal in a chronic thrombus is typically isointense on T1WI and isointense or hyperintense on T2WI, but significant variability in thrombus signal intensity exists. The signal intensity may be similar to that of very slowly moving oxygenated blood. On images acquired after gadolinium administration, marked contrast enhancement may be observed that resembles the enhancement typically seen in a normal sinus which is presumably secondary to an organized thrombus with intrinsic vascularization, as well as to slow flow in dural and intrathrombus collateral channels. Contrast enhancement of the sinus on MR images does not definitively indicate patency, and venography usually is necessary for a definitive diagnosis [10, 12].

Gradient echo (GE) and susceptibility-weighted sequences (SWI) are useful in showing blooming artefacts within the thrombosed sinus in the deoxy- and methaemoglobin stages of thrombus evolution. This can be helpful particularly in the acute stage where the thrombus is hypointense on T2WI. This sequence is particularly useful in imaging thrombosed cortical veins, which can be difficult to be diagnosed on other sequences. It is important to note that arterial flow voids, intracranial calcification, and the bony calvarium can also induce susceptibility artefact. This is of particular relevance around the transverse sinuses, jugular bulb, and sigmoid sinus where this can mimic thrombus blooming [10, 13].

Indirect signs of CVST represent changes in the brain parenchyma as a consequence of the venous flow obstruction and are present in about 40–60% of cases of CVST [1]. Those changes may be located near the drainage of the involved sinus, therefore may be bilateral or paramedian due to midline location of venous sinuses and major cerebral veins.

Venous ectasia, prominent medullary veins, and enhancement of the falx cerebri and tentorium are imaging findings that can develop secondary to increased retrograde pressure and should raise suspicion of CVT. Sulcal effacement can be one of the earliest findings of venous ischaemia, followed by diffuse parenchymal oedema, decreased grey and white matter differentiation or ventricular effacement [1, 10]. Less frequent findings are gyral enhancement, which may extend to the white matter, and tentorial and leptomeningeal enhancement.

Infarct-related lesions that do not follow usual arterial vascular territories or intracranial haemorrhage are revealed on CT or MRI in a case of CVST.

Vasogenic oedema in venous infarct develops secondary to elevated retrograde venous pressure; and it is seen as hyperintense areas on DWI with high ADCs, in comparison to cytotoxic oedema which appears as lesion with low ADCs. Vasogenic and cytotoxic oedema may coexist resulting in heterogeneous pattern at diffusion weighted MRI and heterogeneous ADCs [1].

Venous infarcts can undergo haemorrhagic transformation or presents with intracranial haemorrhages, including intraparenchymal haematoma and subarachnoid haemorrhage typically within the cerebral convexity. Parenchymal haemorrhage is observed in 30–35% of cases, typically in the cortex and extending subcorti-

cally [14]. Haemorrhages in the frontal and parietal lobes are characteristic of superior sagittal sinus thrombosis, whereas those in the temporal and occipital lobes are more characteristic of transverse sinus thrombosis [1].

CVST could involve one or more small cortical draining veins. In superior sagittal sinus thrombosis involvement of cortical draining vein on superolateral surfaces of the hemispheres results in variable amount of oedema and petechial haemorrhage involving cortex and subcortical white matter.

Contrast-enhanced MR venography and CT venography are the best techniques for detecting CVST, and MR venography is the technique of choice for assessing recanalization after treatment. Complete recanalization is achieved more often in patients in whom CSVT affects the superior sagittal or the straight sinus than in whom it affects the transverse sinus or sigmoid sinus, although complete recanalization is not necessary for clinical recovery [1]. With the widespread usage of CTV and MRV, digital subtraction angiography is seldom required for the diagnosis of CVST and largely unavailable outside of tertiary institutions [10].

The patient had clinical presentation that did not rose suspicion of CVST with neurologist. Since she had a high blood pressure and acute intracerebral haematoma was reported on CT, at first the neurologist did not ask for further diagnostic work-up. On head CT performed in the EHD small, oval extra-axial hyperdense lesion adjacent to left middle frontal gyrus representing thrombosed, dilated cortical vein was not reported (Fig. 23.1d–f). Venous sinuses did not seem hyperdense on non-enhanced CT. Subcortical haematoma in the left frontal gyrus was not on typical location for a hypertensive haematoma. MRI of the brain performed 7 days after the CT revealed progression of vasogenic oedema and dilated medullay veins (Figs. 23.2 and 23.3). Since there was no filling defect within venous sinuses on post-contrast T1 MPRAGE sequence (Fig. 23.3g–i), particularly in superior sagittal sinus, radiologist did not check signal intensities in the sinuses on non-contrast sequences, especially on T2WI (Fig. 23.3b, c), which resulted in completely misunderstanding of changes visible on MRI, which were typical for a CVST. It was obvious from the radiologist MRI report, as I have already mentioned in the first part of the chapter.

Blood flow in the dural sinuses is seen as a flow void, especially with T2WI and FLAIR sequences. When there is an absence of flow void or altered signal intensity in the dural sinus, the possibility of CVST must be investigated, although slow or turbulent flow can mimic CVT. When MRI was revised, all signs indicating CVST were there: no evidence of flow void on T2WI (Fig. 23.3b, c) and no evidence of flow within the sinus on MRV (Fig. 23.3d–f) which was hyperintense on T2WI (Fig. 23.3b, c), contrast in the sinus without intraluminal filling defect on T1 MPRAGE (Fig. 23.3g–i), vasogenic oedema in territories that do not respect arterial boundaries, parenchymal haematoma. Nodular contrast enhancement within the vasogenic oedema in the left temporal lobe "seduced" radiologist in a way and haemorrhagic metastases were suspected.

Cerebrovascular events may be the first clinical manifestations in patients with underlying malignancy or may develop subsequently during the course. Systemic thrombosis like deep vein thrombosis or pulmonary embolism is well recognized in cancer patients, although cerebral venous thrombosis is uncommon in cancer but could arise in a case of direct tumour compression, tumour invasion of cerebral sinuses, the hypercoagulable state associated with cancer, or the chemotherapeutic side effects. CVST has been reported to be associated with squamous cell cervical cancer, non-Hodgkin's lymphoma, and breast cancer. In a case of this patient, perivascular infiltration in a lymphoma was mentioned in the MRI report as a less possible differential diagnosis [15].

Normal structures and variants can mimic CVT and radiologist who reports CT or MRI

findings should forget about it. I have already mentioned increased attenuation of the dural sinuses at non-contrast CT in patients who are dehydrated, have high haematocrit values or have subarachnoid or subdural haemorrhages. In such cases, it is important to compare the attenuation of the venous sinuses and that of the arteries in both ides, because in cases of physiologic increase, the arteries also are hyperattenuating. Hypoplasia or atresia of the transverse sinuses occur frequently and may mimic a lack of flow in the sinus at non-enhanced MR venography. The right transverse sinus is larger in 60% of cases, causing a false cord sign on CT. Normal variant of a high or asymmetric bifurcation of the superior sagittal sinus could be a source of confusion representing a false empty delta sign. The transverse, superior sagittal and straight sinus are particularly rich in arachnoid (Pacchionian) granulations which are normal structures that protrude into the lumina of the venous sinuses, and thus can mimic thrombus. Arachnoid granulations are usually isodense or intense to CSF and present as focal rounded filling defects in characteristic locations like middle and lateral portions of the transverse sinuses (particularly within the middle and lateral portions of the sinus). These characteristics help to avoid confusion and mistakes [1, 2, 10, 16].

Mortality in the acute phase of CVST is estimated at 4–5% due to transtentorial herniation, or status epilepticus and medical complications, such as sepsis and pulmonary embolism. Total mortality is approximately 10%, with about half of these deaths attributable to an underlying condition, most often cancer [2].

I will not finish this chapter with treatment options in CVST, which in acute phase should be treated in the stroke unit with anticoagulation therapy, but would like to emphasize how important it is for radiologists and neuroradiologists to think of CVST as possible pathology while reporting CT or MRI of the brain, or look for direct and indirect signs of CVST while conducting those imaging procedures in doubtful or unusual cases.

References

1. Canedo-Antelo M, et al. Radiologic clues to cerebral venous thrombosis. Radiographics. 2019;39:1611–28. https://doi.org/10.1148/rg.2019190015.
2. Kristoffersen ES, et al. Cerebral venous thrombosis – epidemiology, diagnosis and treatment. Tidsskr Nor Laegerforen. 2018;138(12) https://doi.org/10.4045/tidsskr.17.1047.
3. Stam J. Thrombosis of the cerebral veins and sinuses. N Engl J Med. 2005;352(17):1791–8. https://doi.org/10.1056/NEJMra042354.
4. Coutinho JM. Cerebral venous thrombosis. J Thromb Haemost. 2015;13(Suppl 1):S238–44.
5. Devasagayam S, et al. Cerebral venous sinus thrombosis incidence is higher than previously thought: a retrospective population-based study. Stroke. 2016;47(9):2180–2. https://doi.org/10.1161/STROKEAHA.116.013617.
6. Khaladkar SM, et al. Cerebral venous sinus thrombosis on MRI: a case series analysis. Medical. J Dr. D.Y. Patil Univ. 2014;7(3):296–303. https://doi.org/10.4103/0975-2870.128964.
7. Dentali F, et al. D-dimer testing in the diagnosis of cerebral vein thrombosis: a systematic review and a meta-analysis of the literature. J Thromb Haemost. 2012;10:582–9. https://doi.org/10.1111/j.1538-7836.2012.04637.x.
8. Ferro JM, et al. Prognosis of cerebral vein and dural sinus thrombosis: results of the international study on cerebral vein and dural sinus thrombosis. Stroke. 2004;35:664–70. https://doi.org/10.1161/01.STR.0000117571.76197.26.
9. Bonneville F. Imaging of cerebral venous thrombosis. Diagn Interv Imaging. 2014;95:1145–50. https://doi.org/10.1016/j.diii.2014.10.006.
10. Ghoneim A, et al. Imaging of cerebral venous thrombosis. Clin Radiol. 2020;75(4):254–64. https://doi.org/10.1016/j.crad.2019.12.009.
11. Guenther G, Arauz A. Cerebral venous thrombosis: a diagnostic and treatment update. Neurologia. 2011;26(8):488–98. https://doi.org/10.1016/j.nrl.2010.09.013.
12. Leach JL, et al. Imaging of cerebral venous thrombosis: current techniques, spectrum of findings, and diagnostic pitfalls. RadioGraphics. 2006;26:19–43.
13. Meckel S, et al. Cerebral venous thrombosis: diagnostic accuracy of combined, dynamic and static, contrast enhanced 4D MR venography. AJNR Am J Neuroradiol. 2010;31:527–35. https://doi.org/10.3174/ajnr.A1869.
14. Ganeshan D, et al. Cerebral venous thrombosis – a pictorial review. Eur J Radiol. 2010;64:110–6.
15. Iqbal N, Sharma A. Cerebral venous thrombosis: a mimic of brain metastases in colorectal cancer associated with a better prognosis. Case Rep Oncol Med. 2013;2013:109412.
16. Provenzale JM, Kranz PG. Dural sinus thrombosis: sources of error in image interpretation. AJR Am J Roentgenol. 2011;196:23–31.

Progressive Multifocal Leukoencephalopathy (PML) After Obinutuzumab Treatment for Chronic Lymphocytic Leukaemia (CLL)

After six cycles of immunochemotherapy for chronic lymphocytic leukaemia (CLL) based on obinutuzumab and chlorambucyl, this 62-year-old female patient started suffering from progressive visual field disturbances. Ophthalmologic examination performed in another facility did not establish anything out of the ordinary, so she was referred to a brain CT exam (images unavailable) which reported hypodensities in bilateral occipital and right peri insular regions consistent with posterior reversible encephalopathy syndrome (PRES). Steroid therapy was introduced and MRI of the brain was recommended to be done (Fig. 24.1).

The lack of adequate clinical information and previous imaging lead to the findings being reported as posterior reversible encephalopathy syndrome (PRES).

Three weeks later, a follow-up MRI was requested (Fig. 24.2). The patient had been clinically stable.

Taking progression and all the other imaging features into consideration, a suspicion of PML was raised. This was confirmed by CSF testing positive to John Cunningham (JC) virus.

Nine months later, there was another MRI follow-up (Fig. 24.3). There had been interval neurologic deterioration—at that time the patient almost completely lost her eyesight and was partially disoriented, unable to care for herself, but no other major neurological deficits were present. Imaging findings were also in progression.

Attempted intravenous immunoglobulin therapy did not yield any results. However, CLL was in remission.

24.1 Progressive Multifocal Leukoencephalopathy After Obinutuzumab Treatment for Chronic Lymphocytic Leukaemia

Chronic lymphocytic leukaemia (CLL) is the most common leukaemia in adults in Europe and the United States, making up to 30% of all leukaemia cases; in Japan that percentage is tenfold smaller (up to only 2.5%). It represents a heterogeneous disease with variable clinical outcome. It mostly affects elderly people, with median age at diagnosis between 72 and 74 years [1, 2]. Clonal proliferation of mature, mostly CD5-positive B-cells and their accumulation in the blood, bone marrow, lymph nodes and spleen is associated with chromosomal abnormalities, namely deletion 13q, deletion 11q and trisomy 12. Further additional mutations may increase disease aggressiveness. The most common is deletion of the long arm of chromosome 13 involving band 14 (del[13q14]), featured in 55% of cases [1].

Many cases are discovered incidentally, by lymphocytosis. There may be palpable lymphadenopathy or organomegaly, anaemia and

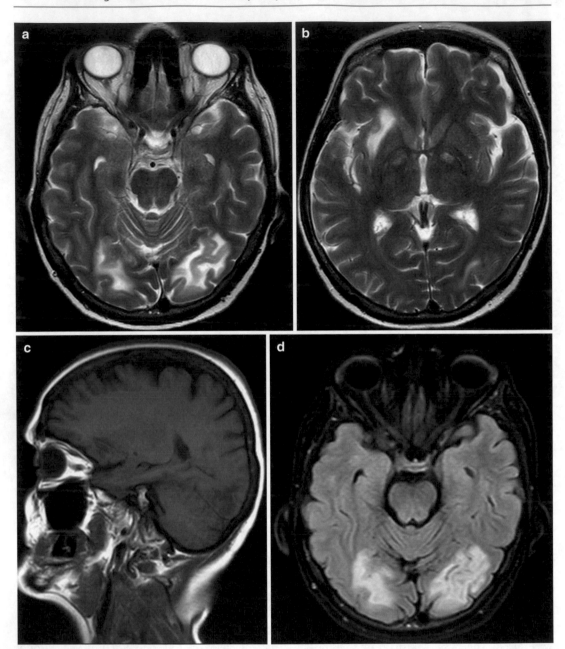

Fig. 24.1 MRI of the brain. Axial T2WI (**a**, **b**), sagittal T1WI (**c**), axial T2-FLAIR images (**d**, **e**), axial DWI (**f**). Bilateral occipital and right periinsular subcortical T2 hyperintensities, hypointense in T1WI, without signifi- cant mass effect. Note the linear diffusion impairment in the right periinsular region in (**f**), denoting the advancing edge cytotoxic oedema

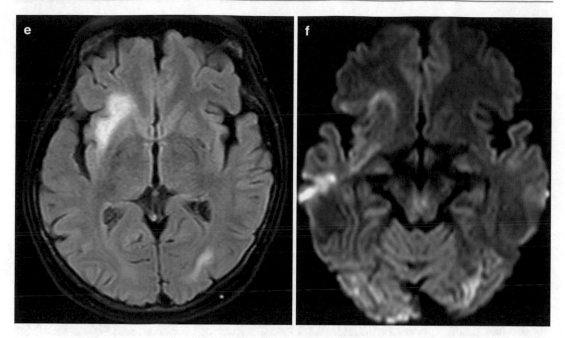

Fig. 24.1 (continued)

thrombocytopenia. Some patients report fever, weight loss and night sweats [2]. Most patients are monitored over months and years for any signs of disease progression before treatment is initiated. The treatment rarely starts at diagnosis [2]. Triggers for treatment initiation include evidence of progressive bone marrow failure (Hb < 100 g/L, platelet count <100 × 10⁹), massive, progressive or symptomatic splenomegaly, massive or progressive lymphadenopathy, progressive lymphocytosis, autoimmune complications, symptomatic extranodal disease, weight loss, fatigue, fever (without evidence of infection) for 2 or more weeks and night sweats for more than a month.

CLL may be treated by chemotherapy, targeted therapy or combination of the two (chemoimmunotherapy), bone marrow/stem cell transplantation, radiation therapy and occasionally surgery (splenectomy).

Obinutuzumab is a monoclonal anti-CD20 antibody used in targeted immunotherapy and immunochemotherapy. CD20 is an activated, glycosylated phosphoprotein expressed on the surface of mature B-cells.

Monoclonal antibodies (MAB) such as obinutuzumab, used in the treatment of lymphoproliferative disorders and autoimmune diseases, bring increased risk of reactivation of latent John Cunningham polyomavirus (JCV) causing progressive multifocal leukoencephalopathy (PML). PML is a severe demyelinating disease with no effective treatment available, frequently fatal. Formerly it was predominantly seen in HIV-positive patients. As for MAB, the highest incidence of PML was seen in patients treated with

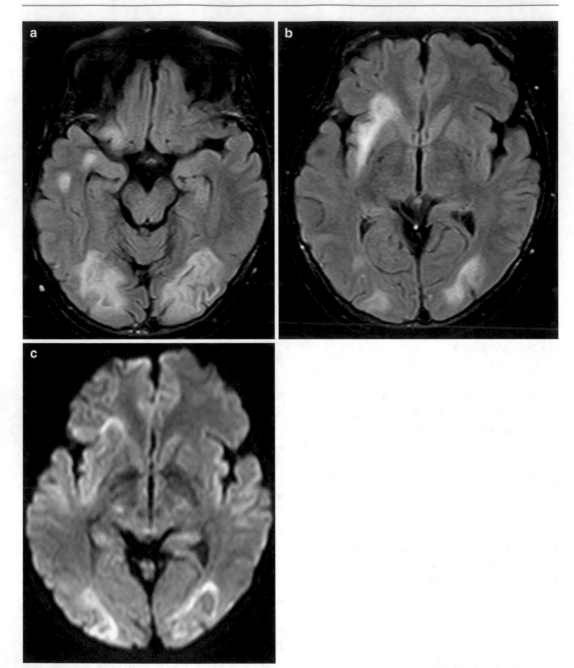

Fig. 24.2 Follow-up MRI of the brain, 3 weeks after the first brain MRI exam. Axial T2-FLAIR (**a**, **b**) and DW image (**c**), demonstrating progression of subcortical lesions to the right-sided temporal lobe

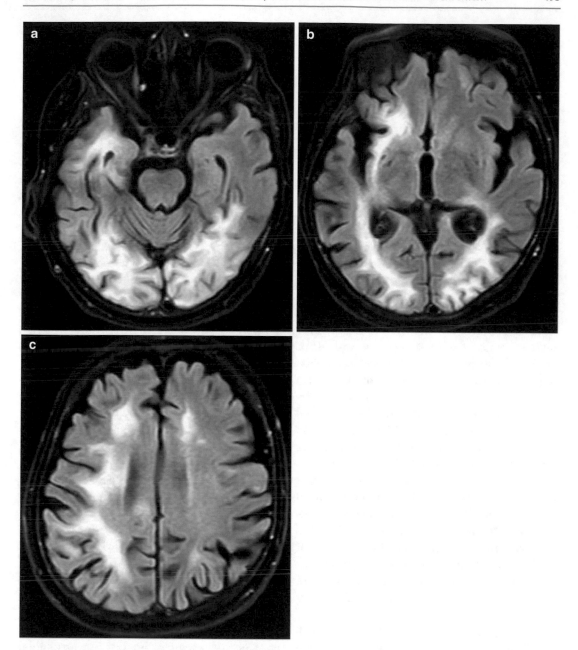

Fig. 24.3 Follow-up MRI exam of the brain, 9 months after the initial MRI. Axial T2-FLAIR images (**a**–**c**). Evidence of asymmetrical progression of the demyelinating subcortical PML lesions—more in the right cerebral hemisphere. There is atrophy of the affected white matter

natalizumab (1 in 1000) and rituximab (1 in 32,000) [3]. Obinutuzumab, being a relatively new medication, was not reported to cause PML until now.

JCV is ubiquitous, found in 50–70% of healthy population; it enters the body via tonsils or gastrointestinal tract in childhood and remains in a latent state in kidneys, tonsils, bone marrow, spleen, lymph nodes, lungs and brain. Cell-mediated immunity keeps the virus under control. In case of immunosuppression or elimination of B-cells (as in CLL immunotherapy), it may reactivate.

If PML is suspected, a thorough neurological examination is important, followed by imaging and laboratory testing. Bear in mind that, although in rare cases, CLL itself may spread to CNS, and most cases are asymptomatic at first. Clinical features of PML are diverse, usually include motor weakness, gait abnormalities, visual field disturbances, aphasia and incoordination [3, 4]. One-third to one-half of the patients demonstrate cognitive and behavioural abnormalities. Seizures, sensory loss, headache and diplopia are less frequent. Visual deficits are caused by involvement of optic radiations rather than optic nerves. Neurologic deficits may be multiple or monofocal [4]. EEG demonstrates focal activity slowing [3]. CSF may contain increased quantity of protein and cells, viral antigen and DNA and lymphocytes containing viral material. The main histopathologic feature of PML are inclusions within virus-infected swollen oligodendrocytic nuclei, often at the periphery of lesions, and large astrocytes with prominent processes and possible multiple nuclei.

On imaging, virtually any area of the brain may be involved. Spinal cord involvement is very rare, although it has been reported in pathologic specimens [4]. It is very important to provide clinical and laboratory information before imaging because of frequent non-specific symptoms and similar, more frequent imaging pathology. As the lesions represent progressive demyelination, they are sited in the white matter (supratentorial in most cases), but histological analyses confirmed cortical involvement in 50% of early PML and 71% of PML-IRIS (immune reconstitution

inflammatory syndrome) which may also be seen on MRI, all lesions with subcortical base [5]. On CT, lesions resemble vasogenic oedema as they present as patchy areas of low attenuation limited to the white matter [6]. MRI is the imaging method of choice, demonstrating T2WI-hyperintense, T1WI-hypointense, asymmetrical multifocal lesions, usually in parietal and occipital lobes, corpus callosum and cerebellum. Central microcysts of very high T2 signal may be seen. ADC values are high internally but low at the narrow advancing edge of active lesion where incomplete T1-hyperintense rim may also be seen [5, 6]. Haemorrhage is highly unusual. Classic PML lesions do not enhance, while PML-IRIS lesions show peripheral enhancement and/or mass effect. MRS demonstrates reduced NAA and increased choline and lactate levels. Perfusion analysis shows low rCBV. There is atrophy of the affected white matter in advanced chronic stage of disease [6].

Differential diagnoses include HIV encephalopathy (diffusely T2-hyperintense white matter, atrophy, MRS with mild NAA and choline discrepancy, without a lactate peak), PRES (usually posterior, symmetric, specific clinical history), ADEM (usually enhance, clinical history); early MS and PML lesions may be similar, but periventricular distribution favours MS over PML.

All patients treated with monoclonal antibodies should be monitored for CNS symptoms and thoroughly examined for PML if they occur. PML is a disease with low incidence but often fatal outcome. Current prevention and treatment focus on immune reconstitution, restoration of immune response to JC virus infection and suppression of eventual immune reconstitution inflammatory syndrome. A successful anti-JCV drug candidate should demonstrate in vitro activity against JCV, ability to cross the blood–brain barrier and possess an acceptable toxicity profile. Immune response modulators increase general immune system responses to viral infection, but in patients with chronic bone marrow depression like in CLL, they cannot be of use. Such patients could possibly benefit from passive immunization [7].

References

1. Hallek M. Chronic lymphocytic leukemia: 2020 update on diagnosis, risk stratification and treatment. Am J Hematol. 2019;94(11):1266–87. https://doi.org/10.1002/ajh.25595.
2. Milne K, et al. Chronic lymphocytic leukaemia in 2020: the future has arrived. Curr Oncol Rep. 2020;22(4):36. https://doi.org/10.1007/s11912-020-0893-0.
3. Bohra C, et al. Progressive multifocal leukoencephalopathy and monoclonal antibodies: a review. Cancer Control. 2017;24(4):1073274817729901. https://doi.org/10.1177/1073274817729901.
4. Berger JR, et al. PML diagnostic criteria: consensus statement from the AAN neuroinfectious disease section. Neurology. 2013;80(15):1430–8. https://doi.org/10.1212/WNL.0b013e31828c2fa1.
5. Yousry TA, Pelletier D, Cadavid D, et al. Magnetic resonance imaging pattern in natalizumab-associated progressive multifocal leukoencephalopathy. Ann Neurol. 2012;72(5):779–87. https://doi.org/10.1002/ana.23676.
6. Rumboldt Z. Progressive multifocal leukoencephalopathy (PML). In: Brain imaging with MRI and CT: an image pattern approach. Cambridge University Press; 2012. p. 238–9.
7. Pavlovic D, et al. Progressive multifocal leukoencephalopathy: current treatment options and future perspectives. Ther Adv Neurol Disord. 2015;8(6):255–73. https://doi.org/10.1177/1756285615602832.

Large Cerebral Vessel Vasculitis in Undiagnosed HIV-Positive Patient: Meningovascular Syphilis

In August 2019, a 47-year-old male patient was admitted to the hospital due to recurrent right-sided hemiparesis that occurred during 12 h. Symptoms started evening before the hospitalization with right side weakness that withdrawn spontaneously after 10 min. Right-sided hemiparesis reappeared during the night and lasted for about 40 min.

According to available anamnestic data, the patient had performed brain MRI about 10 years ago due to an episode of headache—MRI was reported normal. He claimed he had an episode of right-sided weakness in duration of 10 min before 7 or 8 years, after which no diagnostic procedures or medical treatment have been conducted. Patient was a smoker: smoked 10–12 cigarettes per day.

In neurologist assessment on admission, mild right-sided hemiparesis was reported. Head CT and CTA of cerebral arteries were performed in the EHD (Fig. 25.1). All laboratory findings, blood count, prothrombin time, C-reactive protein, urea, creatinine, electrolytes and liver function tests were normal on admission.

Because two successive brain CTs were reported normal (Figs. 25.1 and 25.2), brain MRI was performed and evaluated by neuroradiologist.

During the course of MRI and MRA procedures, I have re-evaluated both brain CTs because it was strange to me why changes of the M1-MCA wall were reported on cerebral CTA without evidence of parenchymal lesion. On CT performed on the admission (Fig. 25.1), I have found irregular hypodensity in the posterior limb of the left internal capsule consistent with acute ischaemia (Fig. 25.1b, c, f), old lacunar infarct in the medial part of the left globus pallidus (Fig. 25.1a, d, e) and small gliosis in the genus of the left internal capsule (Fig. 25.1a, b). On brain CT performed the next day (Fig. 25.2), I realized hypodensity of the posterior limb of the left internal capsule was the same in size, but slightly more hypodense and clearly demarcated.

I have analyzed brain MRI and cerebral MRA images (Fig. 25.3) and reported large cerebral vessel vasculitis with acute ischaemia. Afterwards, I have asked myself why would previously healthy middle-aged patient had such changes. I contacted the attending neurologist to discuss possible aetiologies including drugs and HIV status. The neurologist had informed me that the patient was not a drug addict, but was a homosexual, tested for HIV 5 years ago when he was negative. After our conversation patient was retested for HIV and the test was positive. He was also tested for HBV and HCV. hepatitis B surface antigen (HbsAg) was negative, antibody to hepatitis B core antigen (anti-HBc) and antibody to hepatitis B surface antigen (anti-HBs, 4.34 IU/L) were positive, indicating past infection. Anti-HCV was negative. Consulted immunologist did not think that systemic disease was

M. Špero, H. Vavro, *Neuroradiology - Images vs Symptoms*, https://doi.org/10.1007/978-3-030-69213-1_25

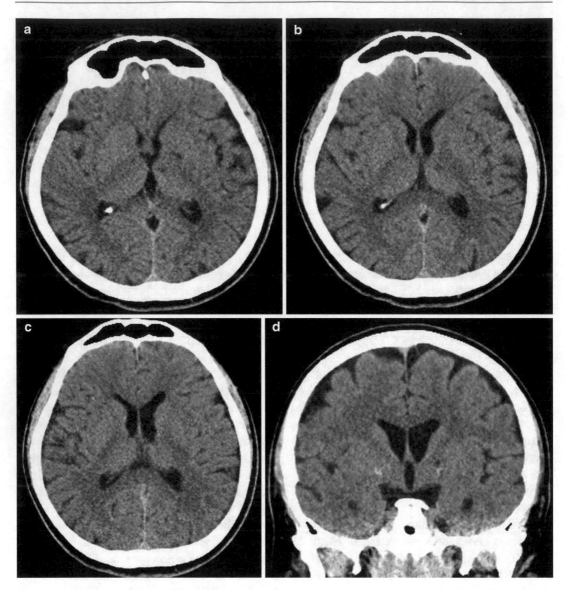

Fig. 25.1 Computed tomography of the brain, axial (**a**–**c**) and coronal (**d**–**f**) scans, and computed tomography angiography of cerebral arteries, axial (**g**) and coronal (**h**, **i**) images, performed in the EHD, were evaluated by inter- ventional radiologist who was on call: head CT was reported normal while middle and distal part of M1 segment of the left middle cerebral artery (MCA) were reported stenotic on cerebral CTA

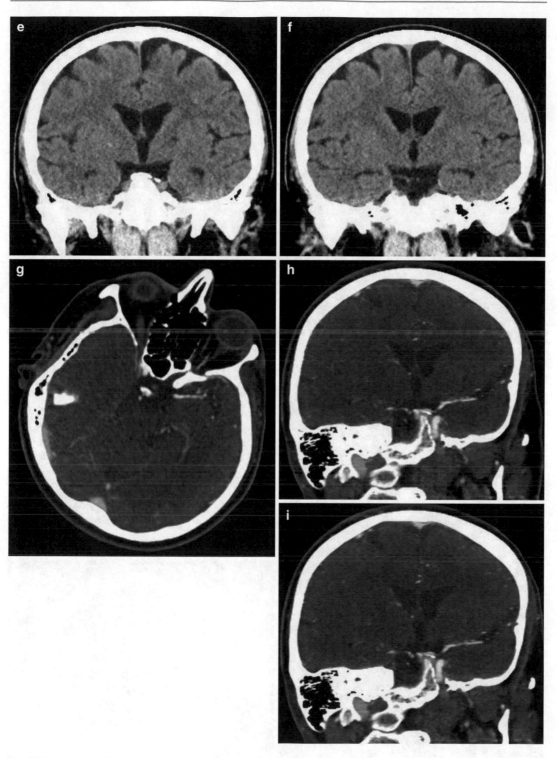

Fig. 25.1 (continued)

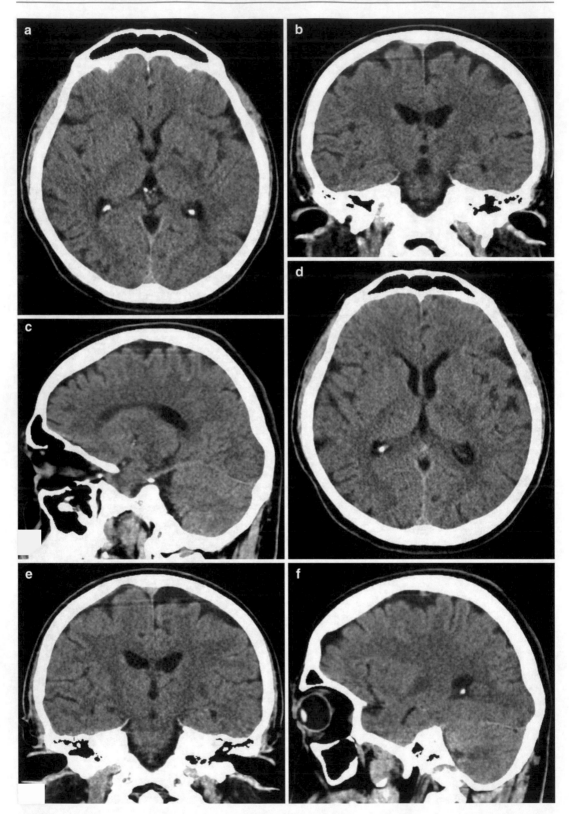

Fig. 25.2 Follow-up computed tomography of the brain, axial (**a, d**), coronal (**b, e**) and sagittal (**c, f**) scans, was performed next day and evaluated by body radiologist who was on call: no evidence of acute ischemia or intracranial haemorrhage were reported

Fig. 25.3 Magnetic resonance imaging of the brain, axial T2WI (**a–c**), FLAIR FS (**d–f**), DWI (**g–i**), ADC (**j–l**), revealed multiple acute infarcts in the left cerebral hemisphere: three punctate acute ischaemia in the left amygdala (**a, d, g, j**), acute ischaemia involving posterior part of the left putamen and globus pallidus and posterior limb of the internal capsule (**b, e, h, k**), four punctate acute ischaemia in the subcortical white matter of the left occipital lobe (**b, e, h, k**), and small acute ischemia in the peri-ventricular white matter of the left frontal lobe (**c, f, i, l**). Old lacunar infarct in the medial part of the left globus pallidus and small gliosis in the genu of the left internal capsule were revealed as well (**b, e**). Cerebral magnetic resonance angiography (3D TOF), axial (**m–o**) images, showed mural irregularities with alternating stenosis and dilatation resulting in beaded appearance of the M1 segment of the left MCA which indicated vasculitis

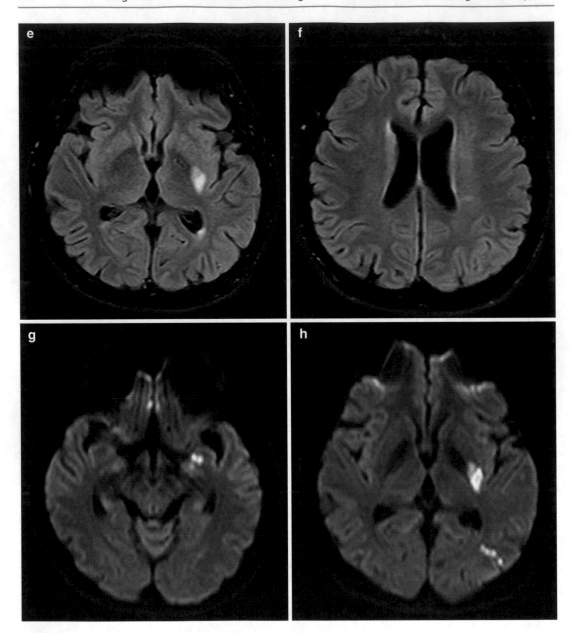

Fig. 25.3 (continued)

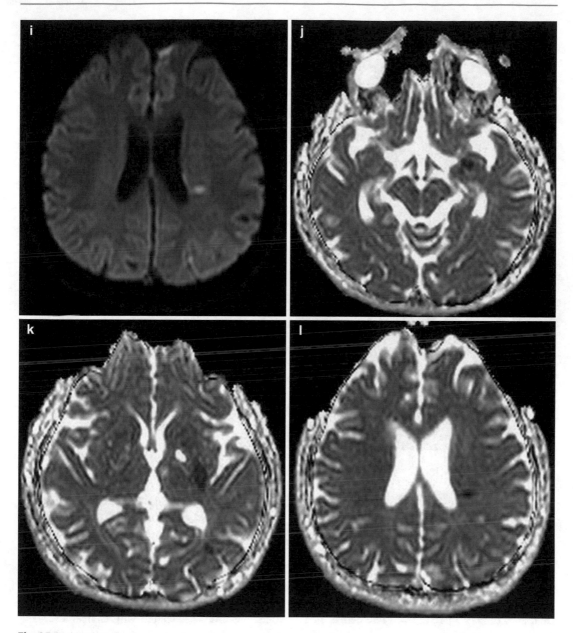

Fig. 25.3 (continued)

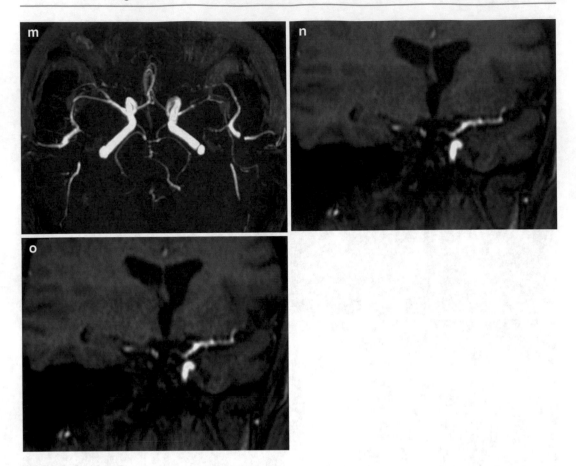

Fig. 25.3 (continued)

the aetiology of the patient's vasculitis: recommended specific tests were negative.

Afterwards, patient was in infectologist treatment: additional CSF analysis was positive for syphilis, final diagnose of meningovascular form of syphilis was made, and the patient was successfully treated for neurosyphilis. Medicamentous treatment of HIV infection was initiated as well.

25.1   Large Cerebral Vessel Vasculitis in Undiagnosed HIV-Positive Patient: Meningovascular Syphilis

Vasculitis of the CNS is a rare entity that may result from numerous causes responsible for the presence of inflammatory lesions at the vascular wall with or without necrosis that lead to obstruc-

tion of the lumen. Cerebral vessels of all sizes can be affected, and the clinical manifestations are highly variable, ranging from focal neurological signs to diffuse manifestations with an acute to chronic evolution. Vasculitis disorders of the CNS consist of primary angiitis of the CNS, CNS vasculitis associated with connective tissue disorders, vasculitis associated with Behcet's disease, and sarcoidosis, as well as infectious and neoplastic diseases [1].

Cerebrovascular disease is common in patients with HIV, occurring in up to 1.9% of HIV-infected patients [2]. In particular, patients with AIDS have been reported to be at increased risk of both ischaemic and haemorrhagic strokes, of which ischaemic stroke is more frequent. The pathogenesis of ischemic stroke in HIV is not well understood, with multiple postulated mechanisms including cardioembolism, coagulopathy, opportunistic infections, HIV-related vasculitis and HAART-related accelerated atherosclerosis, as well [3].

Vasculitis in HIV is generally secondary to lymphoproliferative diseases or opportunistic infections, including varicella-zoster virus, syphilis, cryptococcus and tuberculosis. In patients in whom the above have been excluded, HIV-related vasculitis is one consideration. This has been reported to occur in up to 20% of patients with HIV [3]. While the pathophysiology behind HIV-related vasculitis is not well defined, this condition is more commonly described in patients with low CD4 counts [3, 4].

As sexually transmitted diseases, syphilis and HIV frequently coexist. Among patients with HIV, those with lower CD4 counts are more likely to have concomitant neurosyphilis [5]. CNS involvement is an uncommon manifestation of syphilis, occurring in less than 10% of patients with syphilis [6]. A study of HIV-infected patients by Ghanem et al. identified CD4 count of less than 350 cells/ml and lack of HAART treatment as predictors of neurosyphilis [7]. Lower CD4 counts have also been found to be associated with an increased risk of ischemic stroke.

Illicit drug users (e.g. cocaine and methamphetamine) and men who have sex with men are at the main risk to contract syphilis. After the initial stage, syphilis is a self-limited disease and may go undetected. Untreated syphilitic infection progresses through four stages; primary, secondary, latent and tertiary [8]. Neurosyphilis is a form of tertiary syphilis commonly seen in HIV-infected individuals, occurring in less than 10% of untreated individuals with syphilis [9]. Spirochetes (*Treponema pallidum*) usually invade CNS within 3–18 months of inoculation with the organism [4]. The major forms of neurosyphilis are syphilitic meningitis, meningovascular syphilis, parenchymatous syphilis, and gummatous syphilis. With the advent of penicillin therapy, neurosyphilis more frequently manifests as meningeal and vascular syndromes, not as abnormalities of the CNS parenchyma.

The average latency of meningovascular syphilis is reported to be 7 years; however, meningovascular syphilis can occur within a few months of infection in HIV patients which indicates the difficulty in diagnosing neurosyphilis in patients with HIV.

Meningovascular neurosyphilis is an inflammatory process resulting from the development of typical endarteritis obliterans in blood vessels of the meninges, brain and spinal cord that leads to multiple small areas of infarction. Heubner arteritis is the most common form that affects large- and medium-sized arteries and is characterized by fibroblastic proliferation of the intima, thinning of the media and fibrous and inflammatory changes in the adventitia causing luminal narrowing and ectasia. Nissl arteritis affects small vessels and is characterized by the proliferation of endothelial and adventitial cells. Both the types of arteritis may result in vessel occlusion, with secondary ischaemia and infarction [10]. The middle cerebral artery followed by an involvement of the basilar artery and its branches is the most commonly involved.

Neurological symptoms with little or no evidence of primary or secondary syphilis may well be the first manifestation. Clinical manifestations may vary greatly from asymptomatic to symptoms such as headache, vertigo, seizures, transient hemiplegia, insomnia or behavioural changes ranging from personality changes and emotional lability to dementia. These symptoms may appear from months to even a decade after the primary infection, with an average latency of 7 years.

Typical imaging findings are ischaemic infarcts in the perforator vessel territory of the basal ganglia or brainstem or in the large vessel territory of the middle cerebral artery. Syphilitic cerebral gummas are uncommon. They appear as isolated, peripherally located nodules on CT that appear isodense to cortex and enhance intensely following iodinated contrast material administration. On MRI, they are isointense to grey matter on T1W sequences, usually enhance homogeneously, and are hyperintense on T2W sequences. Cranial nerve involvement, particularly of the optic and vestibulocochlear nerves, has also been reported [11–13].

Angiographically, meningovascular syphilis tends to display focal segmental narrowing and dilatation, resulting in the appearance of "beading". However, these findings are nonspecific and can resemble findings in other medium and large vessel vasculitides, and an underlying HIV-associated vasculopathy cannot be excluded [3, 14].

In the smaller arteries, particularly Sylvian branches of the middle cerebral artery, focal stenosis and aneurysmal dilatation may be demonstrated.

The gold standard for the diagnosis of CNS vasculitis is histopathological evidence of vessel wall inflammation [15]. Brain biopsy is an invasive technique. Therefore, diagnosis of neurosyphilis could be established if there is a syndrome consistent with neurosyphilis, investigations of CSF cell count and protein concentration, and test of non-treponemal antibody as well as serologic treponemal antibody testing are made. Serologic screening for syphilis should be performed in patients with cryptogenic stroke, particularly in those with risk factors for syphilis. The presence of a positive treponemal test should prompt further evaluation for neurosyphilis with lumbar puncture. CSF features suggestive of neurosyphilis include lymphocytic pleocytosis, low glucose and raised protein, which may occur in HIV alone as well.

Neurosyphilis is a treatable disease with a favourable outcome. Treatment of neurosyphilis is the same in HIV-positive and -negative patients and involves a 10- to 14-day course of high-dose intravenous benzylpenicillin. Neurological deficits frequently but not always resolve following treatment.

Many authors state that syphilis appears to be the "great imitator" of other diseases. Therefore, the diagnosis of neurosyphilis remains a challenge, as it requires a high index of suspicion. Recent studies recommend that, due to the reemergence of syphilis, search for *Treponema pallidum* infection should be systematic in young stroke victims [16]. The question remains as to whether the search should include all-age patients even in the absence of a suggestive history.

Middle-aged male homosexual patient with the acute ischaemia in the MCA vascular territory and evidence of vasculitis of M1 segment, who did not use illicit drugs and did not have connective tissue disorder, are highly suspicious for being HIV positive and should be tested for neurosyphilis [13].

Regarding the patient's anamnestic data available in the hospital information system, in the section of "functions and habits", there was no information about illicit drug usage or sexual orientation. However, those information were well known to attending neurologist. As neuroradiologist, I have suspected possible aetiology of multiple small infarctions in the MCA vascular territory and M1 segment vasculitis. The problem was that the neurologist had information about the patient's sexual orientation and illicit drug non-use, but did not think those information could be of interest or helpful to neuroradiologist in reporting MRI and MRA findings. Since the attending neurologist knew that the patient is a homosexual, and I reported M1-MCA vasculitis with small acute infarctions, the patient was tested for HIV and, after the positive testing result, referred to infectologist for further treatment.

The patient also gave information that he had an episode of right-sided weakness in duration of 10 min 7 or 8 years ago, after which no diagnostic procedures or medical treatment have been conducted. CT (Fig. 25.1a, b) and MRI (Fig. 25.3b, e) revealed two old vascular lesions in the left medial globus palidus and genus of internal capsule indicating that the patient definitely had small acute ischemia before. It is possible that those two lesions were small acute ischaemia at the time 7 or 8 years ago when patient suffered from a transient episode of right-sided weakness. I cannot be sure because he might also have been asymptomatic at the time those two lesions originated. It will remain unclear when this two lesions appeared regarding the time of their origin, but they definitely confirm that the patient had CNS vasculitis for some time before the advent of the episode because of which he was hospitalized.

Unfortunately, neurologists do not offer proper or full information about patients to neuroradiologists from time to time, which could be a problem. For me it means two facts, sometimes I have to call the patient again to perform additional sequences or advanced techniques. The second is that I have to search for information myself: I have to go through the patient's medical documentation if it is available, and I have to interview a patient if possible. If I am not successful in a search, then I talk to an attending neurologist. Sometimes I realize, like in this case, they had information, but did not give it to me in advance for a reason only known to them. Sometimes, they did not have needed information because they did not ask the patient or did not suspect disorder I reported while evaluating CT or MRI. Fortunately, those situations are not customary or frequent and my collaboration with neurologists is usually successful.

References

1. Mumtaz S, et al. Central nervous system vasculitis. In: Current clinical neurology: inflammatory disorders of the nervous system: pathogenesis, immunology and clinical management. Totowa, NJ: Humana Press Inc. p. 257–68.
2. Evers S, et al. Ischaemic cerebrovascular events in HIV infection. Cerebrovas Dis. 2003;15:199–205.
3. Jan K, et al. Ischemic stroke in an HIV positive patient: an initial presentation of neurosyphilis. Case Rep Neurological Med. 2018;2018:2410154. https://doi.org/10.1155/2018/2410154.
4. Vaitkus A, et al. Meningovascular neurosyphilis: a report of stroke in a young adult. Medicina (Kaunas). 2010;46(4):282–5.
5. Marra CM, et al. Cerebrospinal fluid abnormalities in patients with syphilis: association with clinical and laboratory features. J Infect Dis. 2004;189(3):369–76.
6. Abkur TM, et al. Neurosyphilis presenting with a stroke-like syndrome. BMJ Case Rep. 2015;2015:bcr2014206988.
7. Ghanem KG, et al. Neurosyphilis in a clinical cohort of HIV-1-infected patients. AIDS. 2008;22(10):1145–51.
8. Krishnan D, et al. Neurosyphilis presenting as an acute ischemic stroke. Clin Med. 2020;20(1):95–7.
9. Hook EW, Chansolme DH. Neurosyphilis. In: Roos KL, editor. Principles of neurologic infectious diseases. New York: McGraw-Hill; 2005. p. 215–32.
10. Pezzini A, et al. Meningovascular syphilis: a vascular syndrome with typical features? Cerebrovasc Dis. 2001;11:352–3.
11. Senocak E, et al. Imaging features of CNS involvement in AIDS. Diagn Interv Radiol. 2010;16:193–200.
12. Abdel Razek AAK, et al. Imaging spectrum of CNS vasculitis. Radiographics. 2014;34:873–94.
13. Ruisanchez A, et al. Role of MRI in early detection of stroke secondary to neurosyphilis in an elderly patient. Neurol Clin Pract. 2017;7(2):12–5.
14. Holland BA, et al. Meningovascular syphilis: CT and MR findings. Radiology. 1986;158:439–42.
15. Cheron J, et al. Response of human immunodeficiency virus-associated cerebral angiitis to the combined antiretroviral therapy. Front Neurol. 2017;8:95.
16. Lachaud S, et al. Stroke, HIV and meningovascular syphilis: study of three cases [in French]. Rev Neurol. 2010;166:76–82.

Cerebral Amyloid Angiopathy vs Primary Brain Tumour (Glioblastoma)

In April 2016, a 65-year-old male patient presented with a sudden onset of altered sensorium, he was a bit confused and disoriented. Head computed tomography was performed in the EHD and revealed intra-cerebral haematoma in the right frontal lobe (Fig. 26.1). Therefore, he was admitted to the hospital. Arterial blood pressure on admission was 145/80 mmHg. There was no history suggesting a bleeding disorder or head trauma.

MRI of the brain was performed 2 days after the head CT to exclude possible underlying pathology. Neuroradiologist confirmed right frontal acute haematoma without evidence of underlying arteriovenous or cavernous malformation, as well as no evidence of a brain tumour (Fig. 26.2). T2*-weighted GRE imaging revealed cortical superficial siderosis (cSS) as a chronic sequelae of previous convexity subarachnoid haemorrhage, indicating cerebral amyloid angiopathy as a probable cause of the right frontal lobe haematoma (Fig. 26.3).

Neurosurgeon was consulted regarding possible surgical treatment. Disregarding the neuroradiologist report, neurosurgeon on his own concluded a primary brain tumour—glioblastoma, was the underlying pathology and recommended surgery as soon as patient condition allowed. Afterwards the neurologist consulted a neuroradiologist, and together they concluded that neither clinical symptoms nor CT and MRI findings supported possibility of a tumour.

Several follow-up CT and MRI of the brain were performed and revealed slightly slower, but complete haematoma resolution (Fig. 26.4). There was no evidence of glioblastoma underlying right frontal lobe haematoma. Patient symptoms gradually regressed.

The patient was without new symptoms and evidence of new haemorrhage until October 2017 when he presented with sudden onset of left-sided hemiparesis. Head CT was performed on the admission to the hospital and revealed small post-central intracerebral haematoma in the right parietal lobe with mild perilesional vasogenic oedema (Fig. 26.5a). MRI of the brain was performed 2 days after the CT due to progression of left-sided hemiparesis to hemiplegia. MRI confirmed acute haematoma and progression of cerebral amyloid angiopathy with progression of cSS in cortical sulci of the right parietal lobe and new one in the cortical sulci of the left superior and middle frontal gyri in comparison to the MRI from 2016 (Fig. 26.5).

26.1 Cerebral Amyloid Angiopathy vs Primary Brain Tumour (Glioblastoma)

Cerebral amyloid angiopathy (CAA) is a microangiopathy characterized by deposition of beta-amyloid (Aβ) protein in the distal cortical and leptomeningeal blood vessel walls.

M. Špero, H. Vavro, *Neuroradiology - Images vs Symptoms*,
https://doi.org/10.1007/978-3-030-69213-1_26

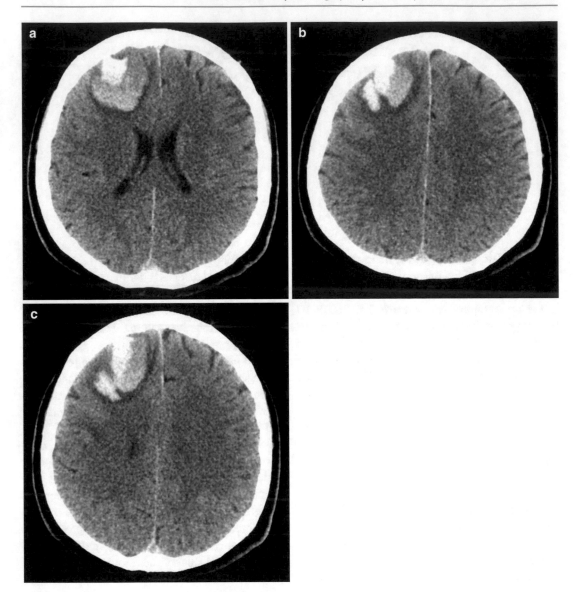

Fig. 26.1 Computed tomography of the brain, axial (**a–c**), performed in the EHD, revealed supratentorial cortical-subcortical acute lobar haematoma in the anterior part of the right frontal lobe surrounded with mild perilesional vasogenic oedema. Due to its mass effect, there was effacement of adjacent cortical sulci. There was no intraventricular extension of the haematoma

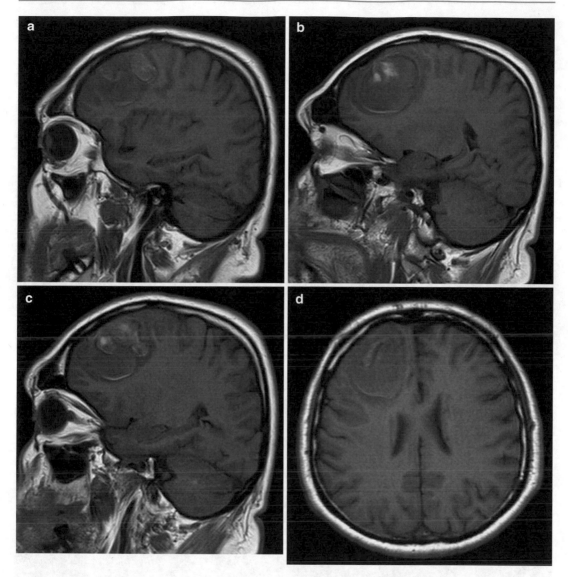

Fig. 26.2 Magnetic resonance imaging of the brain, non-contrast sagittal (**a–c**) and axial (**d–f**) T1WI, axial T2WI (**g–i**) and FLAIR FS (**j–l**), and post-contrast axial T1 MPRAGE (**m–o**) confirmed cortical-subcortical acute lobar haematoma in the anterior part of the right frontal lobe surrounded with mild perilesional vasogenic oedema. Haematoma was mainly iso- to hypointense on T1WI with a few small hyperintense zones, and hypointense on T2WI indicating acute stage of the bleeding. On post-contrast T1 MPRAGE sequence, there was no contrast enhancement. There was no evidence of underlying arteriovenous malformation, cavernous malformation or a brain tumour

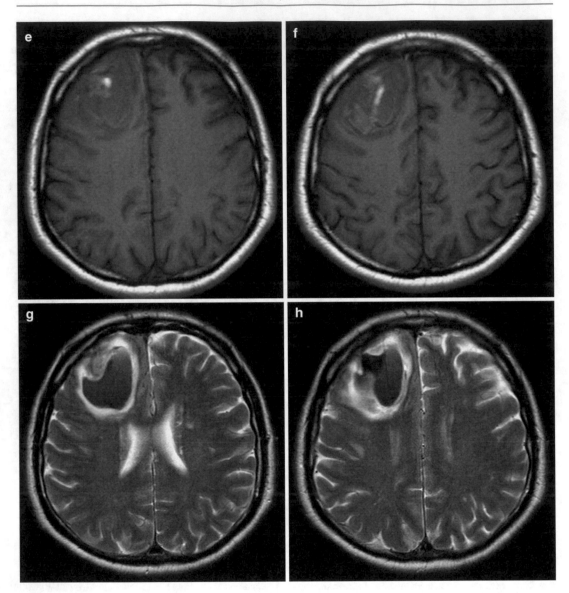

Fig. 26.2 (continued)

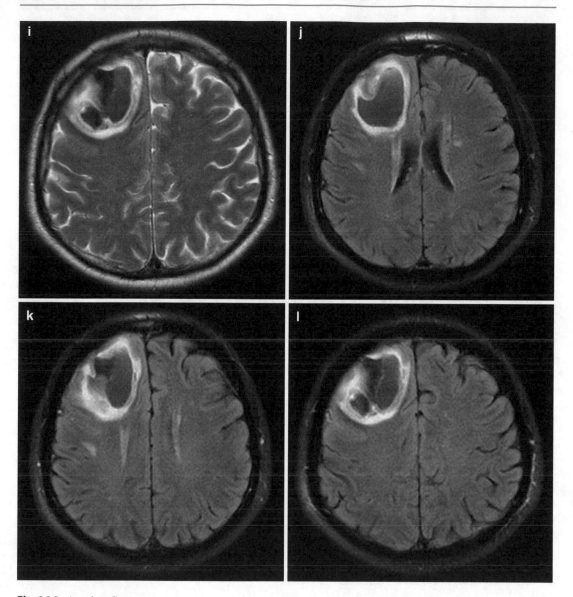

Fig. 26.2 (continued)

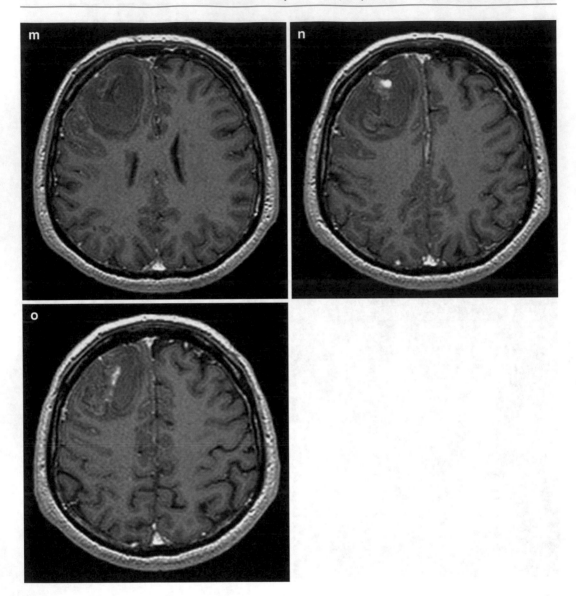

Fig. 26.2 (continued)

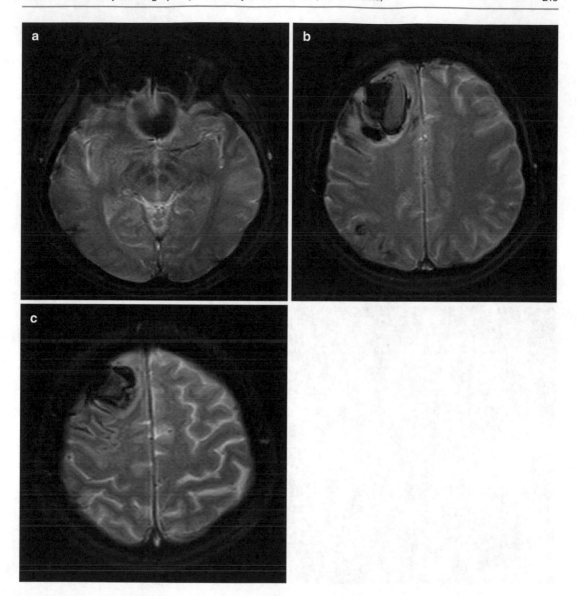

Fig. 26.3 T2*-weighted GRE imaging, axial (**a–c**) revealed cortical superficial siderosis as a chronic sequelae of previous convexity subarachnoid haemorrhage, localized to several right frontal cortical sulci adjacent to the haematoma (**b, c**) as well as in few sulci of the right temporal (**a**) and parietal (**b**) lobes indicating cerebral amyloid angiopathy. There was no evidence of chronic microhaemorrhages in the brain parenchyma

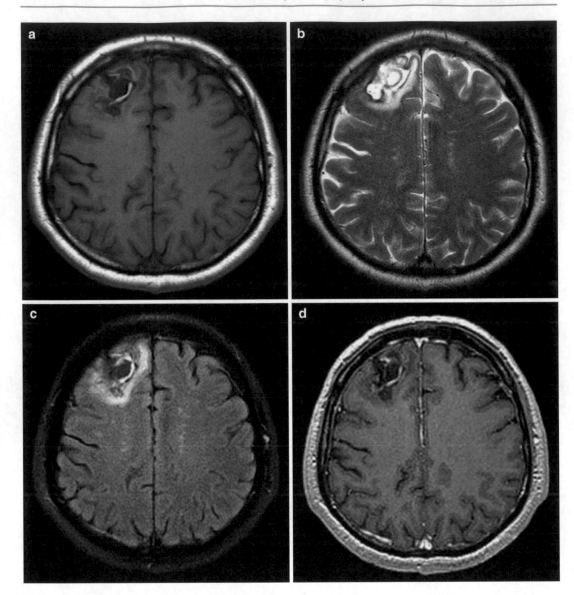

Fig. 26.4 Magnetic resonance imaging of the brain performed in October 2016, 6 months after the initial haemorrhage, non-contrast axial T1WI (**a**), T2WI (**b**), FLAIR FS (**c**), T2*WI (**e, f**) and post-contrast axial T1 MPRAGE (**d**) showed malacia with adjacent gliosis and hemosiderin deposition as chronic lesion after previous haemorrhage in the anterior part of the right frontal lobe. There was no evidence of contrast enhancement on post-contrast T1 images

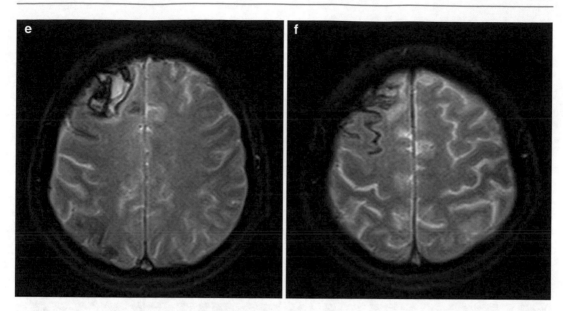

Fig. 26.4   (continued)

Rare familiar forms of CAA occur in younger age and generally are autosomal dominant in transmission. In this chapter, I focus on sporadic form of CAA which is an important cause of spontaneous lobar intracranial haemorrhage in the normotensive elderly and is associated with Alzheimer dementia (AD).

The prevalence and severity of CAA increases with age: it is rare under the age of 55 years, affecting both sexes equally. It is found at autopsy in only 33% of 60–70 year old individuals and approximately 55% of patients with dementia [1, 2]. CAA is responsible for up to10% of all types of primary intracerebral haematoma and up to 30% in lobar type of haematoma [1, 3].

Beta-amyloid is derived from proteolysis of the amyloid precursor protein, an integral membrane protein found in many tissues, concentrated in the synapses of neurons. Different proteolytic enzymes produce Aβ of varying lengths, solubility and aggregation capabilities. Longer and insoluble form of beta-amyloid, Aβ42, is more readily deposited in the brain parenchyma, contributing to the formation of senile plaques and AD, while soluble form, Aβ40, does not aggregate as easily, and can still diffuse through the extracellular matrix [4]. Under normal conditions, all forms diffuse through the narrow extracellular spaces of the brain parenchyma before entering the bulk flow lymphatic drainage pathways located in the basement membranes of distal cortical and leptomeningeal arterioles and capillaries. It is hypothesized that in CAA perivascular lymphatic drainage is impaired which results in elimination failure of Aβ from the brain and its accumulation in the walls of cortical and leptomeningeal small- and medium-sized vessels [5]. At the beginning, Aβ is deposited in the

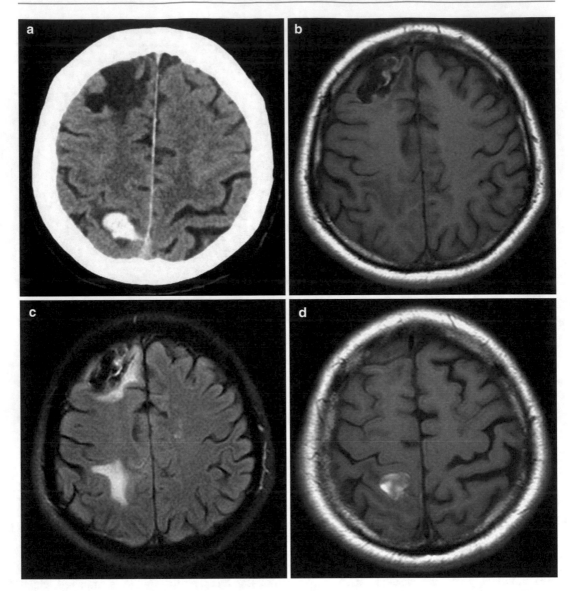

Fig. 26.5 Computed tomography of the brain, axial (**a**) scan, and MRI of the brain, non-contrast axial T1WI (**b**, **d**), T2WI (**e**), FLAIR FS (**c**, **f**) and T2*WI (**g–l**), performed in October 2017, revealed new small acute right parietal haematoma with mild perilesional oedema, and cSS in the surrounding sulci. Cortical superficial siderosis in right temporal sulci showed progression in comparison to MRI performed in October 2016. There was evidence of cSS in the left frontal cortical sulci that was previously not present

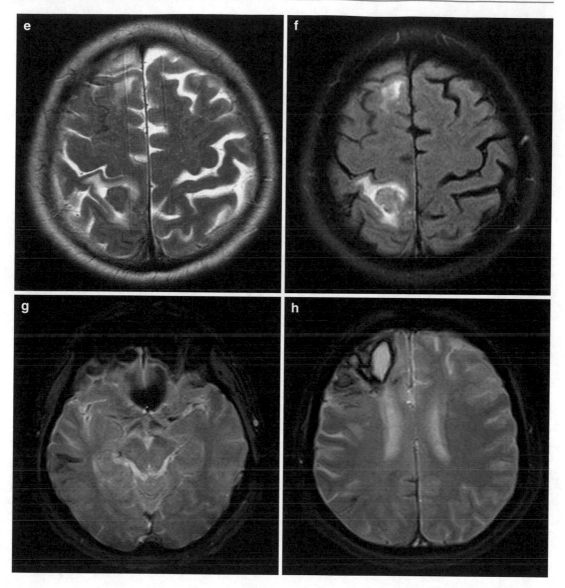

Fig. 26.5 (continued)

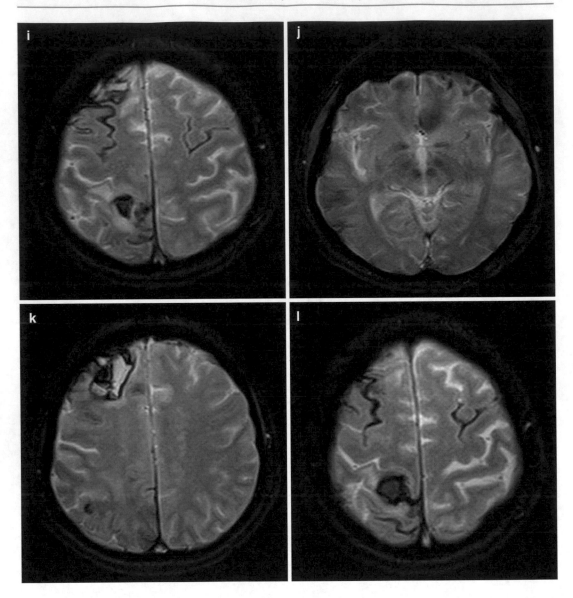

Fig. 26.5 (continued)

basement membrane, while later with disease progression, it involves media and adventitia of the vessel wall. At the same time similarly sized vessels in the deep white matter and basal ganglia are spared. Such structural changes in the vascular wall lead to fibrinoid necrosis, focal vessel wall fragmentation, and microaneurysms, resulting in repeated episodes of blood vessel leakage and haemorrhage, or acute and chronic ischaemic changes due to luminal narrowing at sites of fibrinoid necrosis [5, 6]. The result is a

spectrum of characteristic neuroimaging findings including lobar intracerebral haematoma, cerebral microbleeds, cortical superficial siderosis, white matter hyperintensity, MRI-visible perivascular spaces (PVS) and cortical microinfarcts which are considered to be imaging biomarkers of CAA.

Clinical presentation of symptomatic CAA include stroke-related symptoms due to acute intracerebral haematoma, transient focal neurological episodes (TFNEs) or dementia [5]. Intracerebral haematoma (ICH) in the elderly is the well-known manifestation of the CAA. Specific symptoms depend on location and size of haematoma and include headache, nausea and vomiting, loss of consciousness, focal neurologic deficits and seizures. Transient focal neurological episodes are the second most common presentation of the CAA and could be the earliest sign in CAA. Typically, TFNEs appear as recurrent, stereotyped, brief episodes of focal negative neurological symptoms (such as paraesthesia, weakness or dysphasia) lasting for less than 30 min and may mimic transient ischemic attack, migraine aura or seizure [5]. CAA-related dementia may be slowly progressive, similar to dementia seen in patients with AD, or may manifest as rapidly progressing cognitive decline over the course of a few weeks without focal neurological deficits.

Brain CT scan is the first imaging modality in the emergency department when stroke is suspected due to its availability, shorter duration time, costs, and sensitivity in detecting acute bleeds in comparison to brain MRI. This imaging method provides crucial information regarding characteristics of different haemorrhagic conditions, including volume, shape and distribution. Additional CT angiography is useful to exclude possible underlying pathological conditions, e.g. aneurysms, arteriovenous malformation, fistula and venous thrombosis, which could cause such haemorrhagic complications.

On brain CT, acute intraparenchymal haemorrhage is well-defined, hyperdense lesion surrounded with variable perilesional oedema, demonstrating variable degree of mass-effect. In CAA, intracerebral haematoma is superficial, located at the cortical–subcortical junction, in correlation with the anatomic distribution of Aβ-containing vessels, and lobar in topography with preference for occipital and temporal lobes, but could involve parietal and frontal lobes as well. Such lobar haematomas usually have irregular borders and can extend into the overlying convexity subarachnoid space or subdural space, while extension to the lateral ventricle is not typical. CAA-related lobar haematoma tends to be recurrent in nature, with reported recurrence rates of up to 30% per year [4].

In contrast, deep lobar haemorrhage, most commonly associated with chronic hypertension, typically occurs in the basal ganglia, thalamus, cerebellum or brain stem and tends to be large, with mass effect and intraventricular extension [1, 7]. In rare occasions, CAA-related hematomas can be large and situated in areas of the brain more associated with hypertensive bleeds. In such cases, MRI with susceptibility-weighted imaging (SWI) is the method of choice at differentiating between the two as it detects hemosiderin deposits present in acute and chronic bleeds typical of CAA-related haematomas.

On CT scan, cortical–subcortical intracerebral haematoma without a history of hypertension, sulcal subarachnoid haemorrhage (SAH) or head trauma, are imaging findings suggestive of CAA which cannot be diagnosed by CT alone and require full standard MRI protocol including T1WI, T2WI, FLAIR, DWI/ADC and sequences sensitive to susceptibility effects necessary in the detection of CAA biomarkers. Gradient-recalled echo (GRE) and more sensitive susceptibility-weighted imaging (SWI) are MRI sequences sensitive to the chronic blood breakdown product hemosiderin and are used to detect cerebral microbleeds and cSS as biomarkers of CAA which also represent independent risk factors for lobar intracerebral haematoma and its recurrence.

Cerebral microbleeds or microhaemorrhages are small areas of blood extravasation into the PVS. CAA-related microbleeds have a lobar, cortical–subcortical distribution in comparison to microbleeds associated with chronic hypertensive arteriopathy which are located in deep regions of the brain. Microhaemorrhages are evident on greT2* and SWI MRI sequences as small, 2–10 mm, round or ovoid, well-demarcated low-signal areas [1, 6]. They contain hemosiderin, which is paramagnetic relative to normal tissue and leads to large variations in local magnetic fields and a local reduction in T2*. The signal intensity loss is proportional to the amount of hemosiderin present. SWI, with its unique sensitivity to blood products and haemorrhage, is the most relevant method for detection imaging changes consistent with CAA and is far more sensitive in detection of microhaemorrhages in comparison to conventional T2*GE technique [8, 9]. CAA-related microbleeds were initially thought to be asymptomatic lesions, but there is growing evidence that they are a contributor to cognitive decline. Patients with lobar microhemorrhages are at considerable risk of future symptomatic lobar ICH.

Convexity subarachnoid haemorrhage (cSAH) is a nonaneurysmal SAH, characterized by bleeding localized to one or more adjacent cortical sulci at the brain convexity, without spread to basal cisterns, Sylvian fissure, interhemispheric fissure or ventricles. CAA-related cSAH may be due to SAH resulting from disruption of fragile Aβ-laden convexity leptomeningeal vessels, or due to direct extension of the cortical–subcortical haemorrhage into the subarachnoid space [6]. It can be detected by both CT and MRI. On CT, cSAH may appear as a subtle curvilinear hyperdensity localized to one or more adjacent sulci. FLAIR MRI sequence is more sensitive: acute haemorrhage appears as high signal. Cortical superficial siderosis represents hemosiderin residue in the subpial layers of the supratentorial brain after repeating cSAH resolution and is detected on greT2* or SW imaging as characteristic curvilinear, homogeneously hypointense signal that follows the gyral cortical surface. It is associated with TFNEs and possibly with cognitive impairment, although it is not clear whether this is because cSS is a marker of severe CAA or because it has direct and independent effects on cognition [7].

In CAA, cerebral white matter will be involved because of its vulnerability to ischaemia due to Aβ involvement of small penetrating arterioles that arise from leptomeningeal arteries which are not anastomosing with the end arteries. Those cerebral white matter changes are detected on CT as hypodensity, while on T2WI and FLAIR are hyperintense, spare the subcortical U fibres and do not have mass like effect [6]. Those lesions tend to be distributed posteriorly in periventricular regions and in the centrum semiovale which is compatible with predilection of CAA pathology for posterior brain regions.

In advanced CAA, acute and subacute ischaemic infarctions are not infrequent, occurring in approximately 15% of patient with CAA due to impaired cerebral blood flow regulation in the setting of CAA-related occlusive arteriopathy [6]. Frequently they are multiple and located in the cortical ribbon or underlying subcortical white matter, diagnosed on MRI as small and mostly ovoid or round areas of restricted diffusion on DWI and ADC sequences.

Perivascular spaces (PVSs) are extensions of subarachnoid spaces that surround small penetrating cortical arterioles and venules as they run from brain surfaces into brain parenchyma, draining cerebrospinal fluid to ventricles. MRI-visible PVSs, mainly at the centrum semiovale, associated with other CAA-related imaging findings are suggestive of CAA. In contrast, MRI-visible PVSs predominantly at the basal ganglion are linked to hypertensive vasculopathy implying involvement of deep penetrating small vessels [7]. They are not appreciable with CT, but on T2WI are seen in the cerebral white matter as either small round or ovoid high-signal regions when imaged perpendicular to the course of their draining vessel, or as thin linear high-signal structures when imaged parallel to the course of their draining vessel following CSF signal intensity on all sequences. It is believed that enlarged PVSs at centrum semiovale might indicate impairment in clearance system resulting in Aβ accumulation at superficial cortical and leptomeningeal vessels in CAA [7].

In CAA, atrophy is most likely the result of chronic small vessel ischaemia related to Aβ deposition and is usually seen in association with leukoencephalopathy.

The patient had a larger cortical–subcortical frontal lobe haematoma with extension to few adjacent cortical sulci and typical clinical presentation of frontal lobe haematoma that together with MRI findings were suggestive of CAA. MRI findings were reported as CAA-related changes. Due to good communication with the attending neurologist, neurosurgical intervention was avoided although the neurosurgeon was more than prone to operate the patient because his opinion was that primary brain glioma is an underlying pathology of frontal lobe haematoma. Clinical course as well as regression of haematoma and progression of cSS and later in course of disease haematoma recurrence have proved how right neuroradiologist was when claimed CAA was underlying pathology and prevented, in the case, unnecessary surgical procedure. In rare cases, CAA could manifests as an infiltrative, poorly defined translobar mass like lesion, termed tumefactive CAA, which is hypointense on T1W and hyperintense on T2W images with a variable leptomeningeal enhancement. Such features may be difficult to distinguish from low-grade gliomas or even from lymphoma after administration of steroids [9].

In clinical practice, CAA is diagnosed under the assistance of brain MRI with blood-sensitive sequences using the Boston criteria, developed in the mid-1990s as a tool to both improve and standardize the diagnosis of CAA. The criteria specify four diagnostic categories: definite CAA, probable CAA with supporting pathologic evidence, probable CAA and possible CAA, depending on a combination of clinical, imaging and histologic data [1]. A "definite" diagnosis of CAA is made with a full postmortem examination or according to histopathological findings after haematoma evacuation. According to modified Boston criteria, patients older than 55 years who develop multiple, strictly lobar, cortical or cortical–subcortical haemorrhage, including ICH and CMBs, or single lobar haemorrhage with focal or disseminated cSS, could be diagnosed with probable CAA after excluding other possible causes of haemorrhagic events [7]. The MRI-based modified Boston criteria have excellent sensitivity and good specificity for CAA— clinician should take into consideration that CAA may coexist with hypertension like in our patient [7]. Therefore, these criteria, along with clinical presentation suggestive of CAA, can be safely used to make diagnosis of CAA without the need for "gold-standard" histopathology from biopsy.

Differential diagnosis of ICH includes haematoma caused by hypertension, trauma, bleeding diatheses, amyloid angiopathy, illicit drug use (mostly amphetamines and cocaine) and vascular malformations. Infrequent causes include haemorrhagic tumours, ruptured aneurysms and vasculitis [1, 6]. The history, physical examination findings and laboratory results often allow establishment of one of these diagnoses.

Acute CAA-related ICH should be treated in the same way as ICH due to any other aetiology. If surgery is undertaken, the specimen should be sent for histopathological and immunochemical examination [10]. In anticoagulation-related ICH, appropriate therapy should be commenced to reverse anticoagulation. Currently, no disease-modifying therapies are available for CAA. Thus, attention is directed instead to prevention of adverse outcomes associated with the natural history of CAA, such as recurrent haemorrhages or progressive dementia [1].

References

1. Chao CP, et al. Cerebral amyloid angiopathy: CT and mr imaging findings. Radiographics. 2016;26:1517–31.
2. Masuda J, et al. Autopsy study of incidence and distribution of cerebral amyloid angiopathy in Hisayama, Japan. Stroke. 1988;19:205–10.
3. Ishii N, et al. Amyloid angiopathy and lobar cerebral haemorrhage. J Neurol Neurosurg Psychiatry. 1984;47:1203–10.
4. Sharma R, et al. Cerebral amyloid angiopathy: review of clinico-radiological features and mimics. J Med Imaging Radiat Oncol. 2018;62:451–63.
5. Chen SJ, et al. Advances in cerebral amyloid angiopathy imaging. Ther Adv Neurol Disord. 2019;12:1–11.
6. Sakurai K, et al. Imaging spectrum of sporadic cerebral amyloid angiopathy: multifaceted features of a single pathological condition. Insights Imaging. 2014;5:375–85.
7. Yamada M. Cerebral amyloid angiopathy: emerging concepts. J Stroke. 2015;17(1):17–30.
8. Haacke EM, et al. Imaging cerebral amyloid angiopathy with susceptibility-weighted imaging. AJNR. 2007;28:316–7.
9. Kotsenas AL, et al. Tumefactive cerebral amyloid angiopathy mimicking cns neoplasm. AJR. 2013;200:50–6.
10. Thanvi B, Robinson T. Sporadic cerebral amyloid angiopathy – an important cause of cerebral haemorrhage in older people. Age Ageing. 2006;35:565–71.

Index

<barcode>||| ||| ||||||| ||| | | |||||| ||| || ||| ||| ||| || ||| ||| || |||</barcode>

Printed in the United States
by Baker & Taylor Publisher Services